RE-SOULED

Spiritual Awakenings of a Psychiatrist and his Patient in Alcohol Recovery

WILLIAM GOODSON, M. D.
with **DALE J.**

To Cap & Helen,

Good souls

and

Good Friends —

God Bless You —

Bill

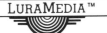

LURAMEDIA™

Cover image by Sara Steele.
  Center two panels from "The Forces of Attraction" © 1984, 1988 by Sara Steele.
  All rights reserved.
Cover design by Tom Jackson, Philadelphia.

Library of Congress Cataloging-in-Publication Data
Goodson, William, date.
    Re-Souled : spiritual awakenings of a psychiatrist and his patient in alcohol recovery /
by William Goodson, with Dale J.
        p.   cm.
    ISBN 0-931055-95-4
    1. Goodson, William, date.   2. Psychiatrists–Alabama–Huntsville–Religious life.
3. J., Dale.   4. Alcoholics–United States–Religious life.   5. Twelve-step programs–
Religious aspects–Christianity.   6. Christian biography–United States.   I. J., Dale.
II. Title.
BR1702.G57   1993
616.83'10651–dc20   93-25392
                                                            CIP

Grateful acknowledgment is made for permission to reprint the following copyrighted material:

Excerpt from ALCOHOLICS ANONYMOUS, reprinted by permission of Alcoholics
Anonymous World Services, Inc.

The TWELVE STEPS, reprinted with permission of Alcoholics Anonymous World Services,
Inc.

Excerpt from COLLECTED WORKS, VOLUME II by G.K. Chesterton. Reprinted by
permission of Ignatius Press.

Excerpt from "Little Gidding" in FOUR QUARTETS, copyright 1943 by T.S. Eliot and
renewed 1971 by Esme Valerie Eliot. Reprinted by permission of Harcourt Brace Jovanovich,
Inc.

Excerpt from MARKINGS by Dag Hammarskjöld, copyright 1983 by Epiphany/Ballantine
Books, New York. Used by permission of Random House, Inc.

Excerpt from MODERN MAN IN SEARCH OF A SOUL by C.G. Jung. Reprinted by
permission of Harcourt Brace Jovanovich, Inc.

Excerpt from THE SEVEN STOREY MOUNTAIN by Thomas Merton, copyright 1948 by
Harcourt Brace Jovanovich, Inc. and renewed 1976 by The Trustees of the Merton Legacy
Trust. Reprinted by permission of the publisher.

Dr. Goodson and Dale are donating
the authors' proceeds from this book
to a halfway house for alcoholic women.

For Houston Goodson and Curtis J.,
who are helping people in more ways
than they ever could have known.

CONTENTS

ACKNOWLEDGMENTS

The contents of the book itself will suggest many persons to whom I am indebted. Their names are not camouflaged in the text, with the exception of patients.

There are many others whom I want to mention in particular. My mother comes to mind right away. It was that courageous lady who answered my timorous request: "Mother, I want you to read this book before it's published because it includes some family secrets. Do you want me to publish it?" Her response came without hesitation: "Bill, you go right ahead. I trust you, and if it helps one person, it will be worth it." Then she read the manuscript and didn't flinch.

Likewise, my sister Pat has been a constant source of inspiration and encouragement, as well as helpful criticism. The rest of my immediate family — Elise, Dorothy, Cindy, Willa, Mary Lou, and Herb — have been nothing but supportive.

And speaking of courage, Dale's family of Mary Lou, Jeff, Brad, and Deb have backed him and me all the way in this endeavor.

Renae Phillips used her considerable typing and organizing skills, not to mention the miracle she wrought, when she pulled the fledgling manuscript from the wreckage of our office after a tornado struck.

I mustn't forget the staff of Crestwood Hospital, as well as all those alcoholics and addicts I have been privileged to treat.

Perhaps Lura and Marcia, my editors, were the most courageous and perspicacious of all, to see in this novice writer's early efforts the making of something I only glimpsed in the beginning. I am grateful for their very personal and gentle guidance.

RE-SOULED

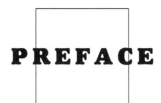

PREFACE

Most people have their own ideas about alcoholics and alcoholism, based on personal experience or on what they've heard or read. Many of you have had first-hand knowledge of addicted persons and have lived with the pain and frustration wrought by the disease. Likewise, many of you have felt the joy accompanying the recovery of these persons.

Psychiatrists are people, too. So I include myself among the "many." I decided that I might have something to say about alcoholics and psychiatrists. I knew that the fragile and, yes, fractious history of the relationship between these two groups left something to be desired. But I had the notion that I had managed to breach the gap and had come to a decent understanding of my role in the recovery of my alcoholic patients. So I thought I'd like to write a book about my understandings, to share them with others.

That's how this got started. Furthermore, I knew that this was a very personal thing with me. I have not been always a devotee of alcoholic treatment practices. It has been a tortuous struggle from medical school to later practice to find my way to a positive outlook on the matter. The changes in me took root slowly, almost imperceptibly, until I was at a point in my own life's struggle when my contact with alcoholics brought about a distinct personal dividend to me. And I don't mean dollars; it was a spiritual matter.

I discovered that participation in the treatment of alcoholics required an appreciation of spirituality in my patients' lives that surpassed anything I had experienced in the early years of my training and practice. And this couldn't be a surface, fakey thing — patients are more perceptive than that. So I had to be at a more comfortable place, spiritually, myself, for these therapeutic encounters to be effective.

As I mulled over the idea of a book about my patients and me, I scrolled my mental file of those alcoholics I had encountered in the past few years. Quickly I fixed on Dale J. His case stood out as the most instructive and challenging of my career. This was, in part, because he was such a tough nut to crack (no offense, Dale). Moreover, he bore the complication of dual-diagnosis, being not only alcoholic but also manic-depressive. This aspect of his case made him all the more interesting and challenging to me. It also promised, or so it seemed to me, to be an illuminating story to tell.

When I called Dale and told him what I had in mind, he was definitely interested; in fact, he already had the idea himself of writing up his story into a book. (He had been required to write voluminous essays about his life and drinking history during treatment, and he hated to see all that good material go to waste!)

We decided that I would be the principal author and that he would contribute material to be assimilated. And, of course, I had his thick office file and hospital records to review. Mary Lou, his wife, also came to some of our planning meetings for input.

What we came up with initially was not what we have ended with. The first manuscript draft was more technical and oriented primarily toward a professional reader. It included the thread of spirituality, but not as the primary focus. Our publishers saw something else in it, something that required major soul-searching on my part. They saw a story of parallel journeys of the doctor and patient: journeys toward wholeness and spiritual growth that matched each other in significance.

If you're looking for a manual on management of alcoholics, there are some fine references I could give you. If you want a how-to book on treatment of dually-diagnosed patients, this is not the place to find it. If, however, you are interested in the nature of the doctor-patient relationship; in the spiritual dimension of therapeutic practice; and, in particular, the changes that can be wrought in both patient and doctor through their encounter, this may be of value to you.

It is a very personal account. I had to decide, with no small degree of anxiety, to explore my life and spiritual development to a depth I had never dreamed when the project first began. It was easy enough for me to decide to tell Dale's story. After all, I'm the Doctor. But to bare my own story, warts and all, was another matter.

I believe writing this book was a good decision for Dale; I know it was a good decision for me.

CHAPTER

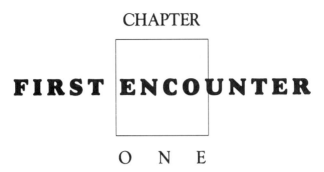

FIRST ENCOUNTER

O N E

"Dr. Goodson, this is Suzanne at Crestwood. We have a new patient for you this afternoon, and I'm calling to tell you about him. He's been in treatment before but seems to be well-motivated. I think you'll like him..."

That was the beginning of my introduction, via telephone, to Dale. His family physician had sent him to the alcohol and drug treatment unit of Crestwood Hospital, Huntsville, Alabama. Suzanne, the screening nurse, had met with him and his wife, Mary Lou, and determined that he would be an appropriate candidate for admission to the unit. And since he wasn't referred to any specific psychiatrist, he was assigned to me as the next one up on the doctor's rotation roster for new, unassigned patients — which can be a chancy business at times, for the doctor as well as the patient. The hospital wasn't a place, you see, where all the beautiful people congregated. So there was always the chance of getting assigned to a crotchety old emphysematous codger from the next county, who had already worn out three wives and four preachers (there seemed to be more preachers than wives those days); or, as in this case, of getting a patient about whom the screening nurse remarks, "I think you'll like him." That meant, as a rule, he was middle-class, clean, healthy, well-motivated and well-insured.

Suzanne then went on to give me the skeletal outline of Dale's history: alcoholic, no other drug abuse, late forties, FBI agent, recent prior treatment, supportive wife who brought him in, history of DTs, depression, hypertension, alligator — his boss. (In case you don't know, the alligator is the prize pet of the chemical dependency treatment field. It has nothing to do with endangered species or ecological apparel. The alligator is the agent responsible for coercing the alcoholic into treat-ment. The image of a gaping, tooth-filled mouth snapping at your posterior should suffice as explanation.)

I had learned over the years how to distill what was essential information to get patients admitted to the hospital and to take care of the immediate situation. Like, any signs of DTs? Vital signs okay? Is the patient taking any medications? Any major health problems? What about emotional state? In Dale's case, fifteen minute checks would be added to the routine detoxification orders because of his obvious depression. No point in taking a chance on suicide. This type of patient is a prime candidate for such a tragedy. Middle-aged, white male, depressed alcoholics are statistically the most risk-prone group for suicide. Especially since Dale was a professional person, the risk was even greater. I would see him later that day, after my last office patient, to check out the situation directly.

While Dale was being assessed by the staff, he was surveying the unit. Actually, most of his surveying covered the part of the unit that lay on the floor between his feet. With his head in his hands, that was the best view he could muster at the moment; and his vision of the world and his own place in it had reached just about that far. He did not feel good. He was probably experiencing déjà vu as he was checked into the place. It probably seemed like just yesterday (it *had been* practically yesterday — only two months earlier in April, 1980) that he had entered his first alcohol treatment center in Atlanta. Now he had to go through the whole rigmarole again, telling his story to a new set of treatment personnel and suffering through the throes of detox (fluids, vitamins, tranquilizers), hoping he wouldn't go through DTs again. He was feeling so miserable he just let them do what they wanted; he was ready to get the next few days behind him. But at least he was close to home this time.

Treatment the first time around, at the hospital in Atlanta, hadn't really thrilled Dale either. This early relapse was clear testimony to that fact. His family physician had sent him there, with Mary Lou's urging and the blessings of his employer. In fact, all who knew Dale had been ready to throw up their hands on him, and they knew something had to be done. They wanted the best treatment available for him, and Atlanta was not too far away. The hospital had a good reputation in the region for being an established state-of-the-art treatment program. This meant there was a high level of professional care-giver, including psychiatrists, psychologists, and counselors. They provided detoxification and rehabilitation services in a twenty-eight day package that was the typical mode of the day. Also, typically, they relied heavily upon the AA Program and employed recovering alcoholics and addicts as counselors. That had been Dale's first encounter with such an apparatus, and he had been skeptical. After being escorted into the facility, all hell had broken loose.

His first (and only, it turns out) case of DTs occurred at that Atlanta hospital, and it had been a doozy. Vivid hallucinations, paranoia, agitation, and terrible tremors invited a round of treatment complete with leather restraints, tranquilizer injections, intravenous fluids, and the watchful eyes of a host of nurses and large male attendants. Through his distorted perceptions he couldn't tell the good guys from the bad guys, but as he cleared over the first two days, he could see they were really rather nice people.

In fact once he regained his faculties, he had looked around and liked what he saw. The place was nicely appointed. Pleasant surroundings. Comfortable.

However, this accommodating frame of mind had been rudely interrupted with the announcement from his counselor: "Well, Dale, you're through detox now, so you get to start attending group today."

From that time on he hardly had a moment's peace. Up at six a.m. for exercises, then after breakfast the day's group meetings began, not ending until late that evening. An AA meeting often finished off this seemingly endless barrage of group therapy encounters, or classes, or whatever they called them. All this group stuff made Dale extremely uneasy.

This Georgia holiday had turned into more than he bargained for. Dale recalls his impressions of those days:

> In the first place, the AA meetings reminded me of old-time gospel meetings. Right away I knew this was not for me. Some of the other group meetings were a little more palatable, but only barely so. One of the things that really turned me off was the expectation that I would spill my guts to this group of strangers. How did I know I could trust them? Some of them were addicts, for God's sake, not like me at all. You can't trust those people. What if something I said got back

to my superiors at work? And, too, I wasn't impressed with the counselor staff. After all, I had a master's degree, and some of those jokers didn't even have a bachelor's degree, as far as I could tell. What could they say to me that I didn't already know? Besides, I was depressed and feeling withdrawn from the whole thing. I didn't take much to heart that I was hearing. I figured I could probably do without treatment anyway, that I could handle my problems myself.

All of this will sound very familiar to anyone privy to the nuances of alcoholic thinking. These attitudes that Dale was manifesting fall within the broad rubric of *denial*, the nemesis of every recovering person. Denial takes many forms and insidiously works its way into the treatment process. At this point in Dale's treatment career, denial was serving to distance him from the treatment team, fellow patients, and the AA fellowship. The bottom line of all his objections could be summarized as, "You can't help me, and besides I don't need any help."

So Dale stayed his twenty-eight day sentence, just putting in time.

That was B.C. − Before Crestwood, before I knew Dale. While he was being inducted into the alcoholic treatment cadre in Atlanta, I was crunching out the daily grind at home. I had recently been appointed the Medical Director of the A & D (alcohol and drug) treatment unit at Crestwood and was trying to learn the ropes of that business while working a general psychiatric practice. My oldest daughter, Dorothy, was about to graduate from Vanderbilt, while Cindy and Willa were mid-college and late high school, respectively. My wife, Elise, and I enjoyed a regular middle-class life. Seemingly no major problems. Certainly no earthshakers like Dale and his family were going through.

Dale and I and our respective circumstances were apparently far apart. Apparently.

Dale was drinking again within three weeks of his return to Huntsville from Atlanta. Though he had promised ninety meetings in ninety days after discharge (a common aftercare procedure), he fell short of the mark, discovering instead a linear regression relationship between the number of meetings per week and the number of weeks post-treatment. It goes like this: first week, three meetings; second week, two meetings; third week, one meeting; fourth week, no meetings. A mirror image of his drinking curve. Back to his old tricks, Dale was very shortly drinking as much as ever. Soon he was to have an unexpected visitor at his office.

It seems his drinking had not been the world's best kept secret, as he had thought. This sort of blind spot is common in alcoholics and is sometimes seen as humorous. We've all seen movie scenes depicting a staggering drunk with slurred speech who is doing his best to appear sober, and who later thinks he pulled it off and got away with it. Along with this caricature are the many more subtle ways in which alcoholics delude themselves into believing their drinking problem is unknown to others around them. For instance, I often hear patients complain that they just can't possibly come into a treatment program because then their friends and co-workers will know they have a problem!

At any rate, Dale's three-martini lunches had made it obvious to co-workers that things were out of control again, and they had reported him to the regional office supervisor in Birmingham. Relaxing in his office after one of those now-famous lunches, Dale was paid a visit by his boss, who presented the facts as he had been told. Dale feared the worst. He knew the FBI was hard-nosed about these matters. He had already had his chance at treatment, and he fully expected to be fired on the spot. And with only one-and-a-half years to go until retirement! What a relief when he was told that he would have another chance at treatment, that Washington now had a supportive outlook on the disease of alcoholism and would like to see him recover. His supervisor had done the necessary homework; all this was prearranged with headquarters. He talked to Dale, then to Mary Lou, and then to Dale's physician. They came to an agreement that Dale would stay in town for treatment this time, and hence he found his way to Crestwood – again a reluctant but submissive victim, quite depressed. And I was about to meet him.

Making a detour to the hospital before going home in the evening was not a favorite pastime of mine. After all, isn't that one of the advantages of being a psychiatrist? Part of the fringe benefits: easy night call, rare emergencies, and clear-cut hours? Get through with your last patient at five, be home early enough to putter around in the yard, especially on a summer day with daylight savings time in your favor, now that's the life! But, alas, such was not my fate that evening as I walked onto the A & D Unit at Crestwood Hospital.

"Dale, I am Dr. Goodson. Let's talk a while and get acquainted."

That's the usual way I get things started between my patients and me. "What brings you here to see me?" "Tell me about your problem." Or, more congenially, "Let's get acquainted." Then things run along smoothly. Unless, of course, I get hammered right away with something like, "Before we start, tell me, doctor, are *you* a *Christian?*" I have always been uncomfortable with that one, particularly since I haven't felt very Christian most of my professional career, and I never know exactly what they mean, anyway. It usually means, "Are you *Saved?*" but they don't generally come right out and say that, and I prefer not to begin the consultation with a theological discussion about salvation. I learned a good response to that question from a colleague, Roger Rinn, who routinely answers: "Does Methodist count?" That type of lighthearted response usually gets a laugh and serves to avoid confronting the question directly.

No, Dale didn't hammer me with anything like that. Like most patients, he was mild and compliant and nonconfrontive. That made the encounter go smoothly, as it does in the vast majority of cases. But I never know what I'm going to find with a new patient because people are unique. That never ceases to amaze me. I am always in for a surprise when I meet a patient. No two are alike. For whatever reasons, genetic and environmental, our protoplasmic masses are endowed with unique gifts of personality that defy all our attempts to classify, pigeonhole, or describe each other. Call it a soul if you will, call it God's way of ensuring our place in the universe, call it Darwinian variation that hones the next generation of species, or call it all of the above, but the uniqueness is there.

Perhaps nowhere better than in the medical field is this individuality highlighted because of the contrast between clinical descriptions and personal encounters. In medical school I was taught the standard textbook manner of describing the patient and recording it in the hospital "admission history and physical." It starts something like this: "This forty-eight-year-old married white male is admitted to Vanderbilt Hospital with the chief complaint of _____"; and then the physical exam begins with, "This is a well-developed, well-nourished man appearing about his stated age..." These are very structured, robot-like exercises that serve the purpose of objectivity, clarity, and discipline in the clinical process. They are also about as exciting as watching grass grow, and they uniformly tell nothing of the flavor of the patient's uniqueness. But that would take a novel-size write-up to accomplish, and the medical records department might complain. So we go on with our thumbnail sketches and leave the uniqueness for the personal encounter.

We psychiatrists are supposed to be better at this encounter business than other doctors. After all, the neurosurgeon who meets a patient in a coma in the emergency room isn't expected to be preoccupied with the interpersonal aspects of the relationship. Pathologists never see the patient, at least not until conversation is a mute (*sic*) point. Between these extremes and the psychiatrist lie an array of practitioners of many specialties and subspecialties, and within this army of doctors, all degrees of awareness of the importance of the physician-patient encounter can be found. The very word "clinical" has taken on the meaning of a cold, detached experience. Most M.D.s are trained in this mode, and it often takes some undoing to develop intuitive skills and a bedside manner. I have observed that, in the last decade or so, more doctors are paying attention to this personal dimension in medicine, especially in those specialties where competition has become a factor. As marketplace dynamics have descended on medical practice, consumerism rears its head and dictates that doctors treat patients like human beings. Or patients will go find a doctor who does. More and more, we doctors are advised to "be nice" to patients, whatever our specialty.

It sounds so simple, be nice to patients, treat them like *somebody*, not *something*. People deserve to be counted for more than a per-diem rate, or hospital number 00213467. Martin Buber puts it in terms of "I-Thou" versus "I-It" transactions. Many languages mark the distinction by using different second-person pronouns for the two relationships (*tu/du* versus V*ous/Sie*, for example). Perhaps it is not appropriate to expect that every doctor-patient dyad carry the intimacy and friendship implied in the *tu*-relatedness. But it is certainly within the realm of possibility that doctors could care about the whole person and reflect that caring in the dignity and respect afforded the patient. It is even possible to suggest that we could try to like our patients.

True, there are occasional patients who, with hostility and resentment brimming from every syllable, spoken or unspoken, greet me like I am a pariah. I may not like them immediately — the same way it's hard to like a porcupine until you get to know one personally. It's a sure thing, though, that if I don't come to like them soon, I'm not likely to be of much help to them.

We psychiatrists, particularly, are in a position where our attitude toward the patient is likely to be important. After all, the nineteenth century title for a psychiatrist was "alienist," one who cares for the alienated. It behooves me to be of a disposition to find the lovable and likeable in people who may be alienated and shunned in the everyday world. While it is true that most of my patients do not at all tax my capacity for compassion, there is a minority — the porcupines of the couch world — for whom I must stretch myself to like them.

Sometimes alcoholics are prickly. Often they have been coerced into treatment and are resentful. It is not uncommon for the alcoholic to be deceitful and cunning — characteristics that one would not call endearing. Thus, I knew my first approach to Dale at the hospital could be problematic, depending on him.

And also depending on me. What kind of mood was I in? Would I be compassionate and kindly disposed, or would I resent the intrusion into my late-afternoon routine? Crestwood Hospital was not on my way home; in fact, it was two or three miles in the opposite direction, and traffic at that time of day on Governor's Drive was likely to make me either (a) lose my religion or (b) practice my religion. The problem was that I didn't have much religion to play with in the first place. So I had to settle for distracting myself with listening to "All Things Considered," hearing in all likelihood a report on interest rates and their effect on housing starts in small-town America, like Keokuk, Iowa, probably.

So I could have been prickly myself, by the time I encountered Dale. And what if Dale didn't like *me*? Who was this doctor he had been "assigned" to, anyway? Would this one know what he was doing? Or would he be out to gouge an unfortunate segment of society so he could maintain expensive habits (like real estate trusts in Keokuk)?

If, as I have argued, it is important that the psychiatrist like the patient, is not the reverse also true? And what could I offer the encounter that would make this likely? Surely one answer to that question was to be myself. Which was a tall order for *this* psychiatrist.

When I had been in residency at McLean Hospital in Belmont, Massachusetts, my wife could always deduce by the tone of my voice on the telephone if I were with a patient. She said I sounded reserved, with a Southern accent that had mutated from my native Alabama to more like Kentucky, that I didn't sound like myself. I was learning to be a psychiatrist and was still fumbling around with how to make that a part of *me*, at least the me that was available at the time. I was also desperately trying to communicate with patients who, in addition to their schizophrenia or whatever, were also encumbered with New England accents, which afforded little comfort to my fledgling efforts.

Eighteen years later, in 1980, I was a little more accomplished at being myself with patients, and I was on the verge of knowing more about who *me* was. I had been through my own life crisis not long before, an experience that was moving me along toward self-knowledge. I had found that I had something in common with my alcoholic patients: a self-destructive force that had consumed me and blinded me to the larger potentialities of life. I knew that I had to find in my professional life something beyond making-a-living and prestige.

I was forty-four years old, married, with a wonderful family consisting of my wife and three daughters. I was practicing my profession in my hometown, a boomtown at that, surrounded by family and familiarity. I had served a tour with the community mental health center in Huntsville, giving up private practice for the noble venture. But I had failed at that venture and was trying to pick up the pieces. I was spiritually and emotionally dead. I was miserable. I couldn't even take heart from a fellow Southerner in the White House. Jimmy Carter looked straight at me from the Oval Office and told me how demoralized I was. He was right.

Like my patients, I, too, was a struggling person; struggling for a recovery of my own and, at the same time, helping people like Dale. I was beginning to allow myself to learn from patients as I saw them give up the egoism and self-delusion that had prevented them from reaching out to a source of power beyond themselves. Encounters with them were feeling more like genuine meetings of minds, rather than clinical and analytical examinations. So maybe Dale *would* find me to be a suitable sort of person.

I certainly found Dale to be so. The very first minute I saw him, I liked him, mainly because of his obvious pain that was calling out for relief. He was depressed, very depressed. Suzanne, the nurse who had first called me and volunteered that, in her opinion, I would like him, had indeed seen in Dale what I saw that evening. It turned out her comment did not relate to the "acceptability" of the patient, but rather to his submissive and needy state of mind.

From Dale's point of view, the first encounter was a blur.

> I recall little of what happened during that three-week stay at Crestwood, except that I had more classes and more AA meetings in a little white house across the street from the hospital. But my depression did begin to lift as I engaged once again in the rigors of a treatment program.
>
> I also had counseling sessions, which I didn't like, namely because most of them were with Mary Lou, and I wasn't keen about the advice she was getting. The nerve of that guy, telling her to leave me if I didn't stop drinking! Something about a 'three strikes' contract, in which the third relapse would result in divorce. I didn't really think Mary Lou would do that, since she had put up with me so far. And so what if she did? I'd rather have my vodka anyway. I knew I'd be drinking again, though I had learned by now to play the game and say what was expected of me, and I hoped Mary Lou would stay with me. But if it came down to her or the bottle, there was no doubt in my mind where I stood.

Mary Lou's role in Dale's disease is a very important one, of course. If you look at the literature or hear professional discussions about alcoholism these days, you encounter plenty of terms to remind you of this: family disease, enabler, co-dependency, co-alcoholic. Mary Lou had run the gamut of these experiences, from playing CYA for Dale to pouring out his liquor. What a game she and Dale had played: not spin-the-bottle but hide-and-find the bottle. If Dale had put half as much energy into recovery as he had into contriving bottle hideaways, he would have been long sober. It took Mary Lou several years and many psychic bruises to learn eventually the truth about alcoholic behavior — that it can be controlled only by the alcoholic. Pleading, threatening, cajoling, exhorting, all a waste of breath. She was being exposed to these notions in the treatment program and at Alanon meetings while Dale was going through the motions again.

We cut short Dale's stay at Crestwood to three weeks because of his recent treatment experience. Our theory was that he had already been through this once, so he didn't need as much exposure this time. We were to see later that he really didn't gain much, didn't even remember much about his time at Crestwood. So he probably could have used more time, instead of less. Should we have pushed harder for a long-term treatment program at that point? If we had had a crystal ball, we could have foretold that eventually such would be necessary. Years later Dale would be sent to a long-term treatment program far away from home. But soothsaying aside, we gave it our best shot and decided to have a go at outpatient management and aftercare meetings. If we had scratched the surface of Dale's commitment to sobriety at that moment, we would have struck quicksand. But I discharged him with instructions to attend the weekly aftercare program and AA meetings, and to see me in my office for follow-up appointments.

He didn't do any of these for very long.

It wasn't the last that we would see of each other, by any means.

Our treatment encounter would evolve over the next several years, with many twists and turns. It still goes on at the time of this writing. There would be many opportunities for intervention as the drama unfolded. The principal characters would remain the same: Dale, Mary Lou, family physician, and me. Supporting players would include his boss(es), hospital treatment center staffs, and the AA fellowship (cast of thousands). The issues would be complex as the plot unfolded. There would never come a time when I could sit back and relax with Dale; he was to keep me on my professional toes.

I had an opportunity to help change Dale's life. But how could I be sure I was *helping*, not hurting? Psychiatrists in general, and I in particular, had not enjoyed uniform success with alcoholics. Quite the contrary. The Hippocratic dictum, *primum non nocere* ("first, do no harm"), may have been coined with this particular encounter in mind. It's not enough to like the patient and have good intentions. I had to bring something substantial to the table. I had to know what I was doing.

At the same time, I needed to be learning as I went. Dale was to teach me much that I needed to learn about alcoholics. In fact, at that point in my career as an alcohol fighter, I must confess that I was learning as much as my patients. And I was learning it primarily *from* my patients.

From Dale, I began to learn patience, to understand that each patient must be encountered as an individual, that patients don't all fit the same mold. You might say that Dale and I were both recovering: he, from alcoholism; I, from bad-attitudism.

CHAPTER

THE MAKING OF AN ATTITUDE

T W O

"Dr. Goodson, we have an alcoholic patient for you in the emergency room. He's been cleared by the medical resident and needs disposition. Could you come to see him?"

The year was 1964, and I was on call at Massachusetts General Hospital in Boston, sleeping in the residents' quarters. I'm sure the nurse sensed my despair at her words. I had done this before and didn't like it. None of the residents liked it, especially at two a.m.

I knew exactly what I was going to find: a homeless, disheveled male alcoholic asking for treatment — and savvy enough to know that we had bus tickets to the state hospital some forty miles distant, where he would find three squares. My mission (and I had to accept it) was to confirm the diagnosis of alcoholism, certify that he was not otherwise mentally ill or medically unstable, and authorize the bus ticket. Occasionally, I was surprised by a patient who had a home and did not want a bus ticket. Then I had to shake my stereotypic response and attempt to engage the patient toward some meaningful and creative outcome of the emergency room visit.

That was easier said than done because of the limited resources available. The disposition of choice for such patients was to motivate them for outpatient treatment. This was the sixties, before the heyday of twenty-eight day treatment programs. The illness model of alcoholism was on the verge of general acceptance, but pessimism abounded in most medical circles. As a young resident, I found it difficult to work with alcoholics because they would not fit my neat model of outpatient psychotherapy. They weren't well-motivated, they failed their appointments, they lied to me, and they didn't get well. I assumed this was their fault, not mine, so I didn't like them. Soon I didn't even try to like them; I tried to avoid them. Though I assumed the semblance of concern, I knew I wasn't effective with them.

With such attitudes permeating the residents' quarters, it was no surprise when our mentors came to the astounding conclusion that psychiatric residents were not very therapeutic with alcoholics in the emergency room. Patients given appointments to the outpatient clinic the next day were staying away in droves. Hence, a research project was undertaken to see if the show-rate for first appointments at the clinic could be increased. The innovation introduced in this project was the assignment of a psychiatric social worker to the emergency room. This person was to interact with the alcoholic, arrange the disposition, consult with the resident as necessary, and follow up on the case afterward. With this simple change the percentage of kept appointments at the clinic rose dramatically. Why did this happen? Because the social worker was a benevolent agent, concerned, wanting to do the job. The noxious agent (psychiatric resident) was relegated to a less prominent function, which was a welcome change to all concerned. The "bus station ticket office" was transformed into a meaningful place of encounter for the alcoholic patient. This was my first step toward attitude correction. At least I began to see that the alcoholic could be engaged in a positive manner.

Psychoanalytic psychiatry (à la Freud) was the order of the day during my residency training. Theories abounded as to the intrapsychic and developmental causes of alcoholism. Academic clinicians searched in vain for the "alcoholic personality." Ego psychology placed the alcoholic in an arrested stage of oral development, seeking fulfillment of dependency needs by substituting the bottle for the breast. Theories notwithstanding, things weren't working out so well in actual practice. Alcoholics left the couch as drunk as they came in. Or alternatively, the fifty-minute hour was a temporary hiatus in the day's schedule of inebriation.

Repeated failure of standard psychotherapy to effect changes in drinking patterns brought about an almost universal pessimism in the treatment of these patients. Other treatments such as medication, electroshock therapy, and behavior therapy were equally unsuccessful. We were striking out.

Then we began hearing of success with a self-help program called Alcoholics Anonymous. But, we thought, how could they get well without *professional* help? I recall that Alcoholics Anonymous was often seen as "substituting one addiction for another" or as "treating only the symptom," since alcoholism was seen by most of the psychiatric world as a symptom of underlying problems, not as an illness in itself.

All of this theory and practice was not diabolical or intentionally misleading. In scientific good faith our psychiatric mentors were doing their best, with the means at their disposal, to grasp the meaning of chemical dependency. They were, simply — and with the lens of hindsight — wrong.

Unfortunately, this error engendered frustration and rejecting attitudes in young medical minds. We were throwing away the round pegs because they didn't fit our square holes. And it wasn't just the psychiatrists. Most of the medical community was having similarly unsuccessful experiences with alcoholics. Medical students and residents alike were coming away from rotations in emergency rooms with negative feelings. And there were many, many opportunities for alcoholics to encounter the medical establishment.

Dale was no exception. Over an eleven-year period, he accumulated a total of fourteen separate drying-out episodes, much to the dismay of his insurance company and to the delight of hospital administrators. On the hospital records, his true diagnosis was often camouflaged with "hypertension," "hepatitis," or "angina" to protect the innocent. Such was customary in those days, with good intentions backfiring on the family doctor who unwittingly became involved in a revolving door detox cycle.

Dale had been admonished by his doctor to "control" his drinking and had often been given antidepressants or Antabuse (a drug that can cause very unpleasant symptoms if alcohol is ingested on top of it). As Dale puts it, he found himself fighting two drugs, alcohol and Antabuse. Eventually, his physician realized the folly of repeated drying out and gave him an ultimatum: "Get into treatment or get another doctor." With Dale, like most alcoholics, this came later rather than sooner. Dale's physician undoubtedly has learned some lessons from him, too.

Dale had been seeing another psychiatrist on an outpatient basis a few months before he came into Crestwood Hospital for treatment with me. He had been through the traditional psychotherapeutic approach of talking and exploring and analyzing. This had suited Dale fine, since he could keep right on drinking while he got "therapy." After a few weeks of this, he figured he could find a better way to use his money (namely, booze), so he terminated his brief and unillustrious psychotherapy career. He was fortunate. Some patients follow that routine for months or years, setting themselves up for a load of retrospective resentment when they eventually enter a real recovery program with an empty billfold. I think I was poised to offer Dale a different experience with a psychiatrist.

Since my "ticket agent" days in the sixties at the Massachusetts General, I had come a long way. After a brief stint in private practice in Huntsville, Alabama, my home town, I had gone on to accept a position with a local community mental health center. Faster than you could say "Federal Grant," we were birthing new programs: emergency, inpatient, day treatment, aftercare, satellite clinics, all with the purpose of obviating the need for institutions and taking the burden off city hall and the courthouse. Soon it was impressed upon me *which* burden was the most odious – the public inebriate – along with the expectation that we were to do something about it. Though we weren't Skid Row or the Bowery, our community had its share of such problems. There were dozens of repeat offenders, the drunk tank at the city jail, the DUI offender, and a host of other presentations of the alcoholic to the court system. And the powers-that-be welcomed a hand from the mental health establishment.

I knew I wasn't up to the task. I had no idea what to do. Humility came in bucketfuls in the public mental health business!

Circa 1970, the awful truth was out: as in the Case of the Benevolent Social Worker, there was growing evidence that people other than psychiatrists could help people who needed help. There was also a rumor that nonprofessionals could be agents of therapeutic change. And worst of all, it was being said that alcoholics could help other alcoholics!

In my case I was ready to buy into these heresies. A mental health center psychiatrist learns to be practical. I learned to do what worked and to do it within the budget.

Enter Bob R.

He was within our budget, so we brought him on board to direct our alcoholism services. Bob was a recent career Army retiree who had worked his way up the ranks to Major. Along the way he had also tried to work his way *down* the ranks by drinking at every stool in every bar at every military post to which he was assigned. Sweet ol' Bob (or SOB, as he affectionately refers to himself) ended his twenty-five year career on a high note, however, by consorting with AA members instead of barroom buddies for the last eight years of his duty. One of the mental health center board members, an AA advocate himself, knew Bob and thought he would make a good alcoholism fighter.

At first it was hard for me to understand just what our board member saw in Bob. He would have to be described as a crusty, rough-hewn type of guy. He sure didn't use fancy words, and four letter ones were more his stock in trade. Plus, he smoked the worst smelling Italian cigars one could imagine. What did this erstwhile Army officer have to offer? It turned out that his credentials were as follows: (a) eight years' sobriety in AA, (b) administrative experience (Read: understands the need for paperwork), (c) a sense of humor, and (d) a desire not to vegetate his retirement years away.

I learned many things from Bob, though he never seemed to teach. You must know what I mean. Most of us have been blessed from time to time with the presence of people who teach by example. If we stick around them long enough, something comes off on us, and we hardly notice it until it happens. Maybe Bob came by that gift naturally, or maybe he adopted it from the AA tradition of recruiting through "attraction, rather than promotion." That is, AA doesn't advertise or proselytize, but through word of mouth and the sober example of its devotees, it attracts members to its ranks. Bob emanated that sort of presence — when the cigar smoke didn't mask it.

The more Bob influenced me, the more I put away some of my academic precepts. He had a way of cutting to the core. For instance, when discussing the genetics of alcoholism, he would capsulize the discussion with, "Shake any family tree, and out falls a drunk." Similarly, when we wrestled with the often frustrating process of motivating patients for treatment, he might deliver, "You plant some seeds, stir in manure, and wait." Even more graphically, he often characterized an alcoholic's attempt to stay sober by willpower alone as being "like eating a box of Ex-Lax and then trying to sit through a church service." Salty humor has a way of taking the sting out of some of the miseries of this business! More importantly, I saw that alcoholics could laugh at themselves as they progressed in recovery.

But all seriousness aside, as Groucho said, I also was learning from Bob my first lessons in AA-ology. I was getting my first glimpse of the power of that fellowship. It seemed mysterious to me then, this "Program": as in "you're not working your Program" or "the Program teaches that..." The basis of the Program, I found, was the Big Book, as it was called. This bible of AA, entitled simply, *Alcoholics Anonymous*, was a book I glanced at when Bob first showed it to me in 1971 and then put aside, not to resurrect a serious reading of it for many years. I was content at that point to wallow in the mystery and not subject a good thing to intense scrutiny.

Not that I wasn't curious about how the Program worked. I knew

that the Twelve Steps were important, with their "God of my understanding" and "fearless and searching moral inventory." Spiritual renewal and humility seemed to be keynotes, but my scientific mind had
difficulty with all of this. Having been schooled in the physical and
psychological sciences as a medical student, I had done best with
treatment concepts such as stabilizing heart rate and rhythm, balancing
electrolytes in the blood, or modifying neurotransmitters with drugs.
Even we psychiatrists have enjoyed a rapprochement with scientific
medicine, given the breakthroughs in brain chemistry and physiology
of the past two decades. We have elbowed our way alongside medical
colleagues as *real* doctors, wielding our prescription pads with the best
of them. So how was I in this milieu supposed to fathom the murky
depths of alcoholic recovery and accept its unscientific tenets and
spiritual dimensions? I decided to try to figure this Program out, to see
if I could make some sense out of this enigmatic self-help approach.

For starters, I was attracted to the systematic order of the Twelve
Steps, so that's where I began my inquiry. I wanted to know *which* step
was the *key* one. Was it Step 1, acceptance? Step 3, turning things over
to God? Step 8, making amends to others? When I would ask a
recovering person that question, I usually drew a blank. I became
aware that it wasn't that simple, that I was asking the wrong question.
It wasn't *one* of the steps at all. I was trying to treat this like pneumonia:
Which antibiotic is the right one for this bacterium? Not only was I
narrow in attempting to isolate the steps, but also in placing all the
emphasis on steps in the first place. So it was back to the drawing board.
It was hard to get a straightforward answer from AA members as to
what the Program was all about. The more I probed, the more nebulous
it became, like picking up mercury. It reminded me of my youthful

experience in Demolay, the Masonic-like organization for young men. There was a lot of secrecy in the rituals and teachings; and nonmembers, I am sure, felt ostracized. So it was with me and AA. Until I decided to look into the horse's mouth and attend a meeting.

Whatever the original reason for having "open meetings," they surely serve the purpose of demystifying the Program for us uninitiated. Open AA meetings are just what they say — open to anyone. Primarily, they are intended for family and friends of the AA member to come and get an idea of what their loved one is experiencing. I had some misgivings about attending my first meeting, thinking I might run into people who would be embarrassed to see me (and vice versa). But I had a patient whom I had been encouraging to attend, and things sort of fell into place so that I offered to accompany her to her first meeting — and mine.

I met her outside the church school building at 7:55 p.m., and we walked in together, her daughter also accompanying. While I was trying to be reassuring and supportive, I think my mouth was a bit dry. It wasn't my patient I was concerned about; it was me. Would I see anyone I knew? Would I be expected to speak up? I wondered if they would suspect me of being an undercover alcoholic, masquerading as a visitor; or worse yet, a spy checking out my patients.

The outcome of the adventure was most enlightening. First and foremost, I was struck by the honesty of the participants. The very bluntness and terseness of the ritualized introduction, "My name is John; I am an alcoholic," set the tone of openness, frankness, and self-disclosure that was unmatched anywhere in my experience. It was, in fact, shocking — disarmingly shocking. Threatening to some, I am sure, even frightening to novices such as myself, but unmistakably a trademark.

Another impression of this, my first AA meeting, was the warmth and acceptance I saw among the members. Hugs were commonplace, as if this were a big warm family reunion. As I observed, the notion occurred to me that these people *loved* each other. I am sure a bubble with a light bulb appeared over my head at that moment.

"Wow! Zap! They *WHAT* each other?"

"Yes, Bill, while you've been trying to analyze this thing to death, there is a very obvious and simple answer to 'how does it work?' It's a four letter word that makes all the difference. These folks are loving each other into sobriety."

My understanding was deepening. The onion was starting to peel. First, steps; then honesty; then love; then . . . what? Was there a core to the Program underneath these layers? Yes, of course, there was. It was the spiritual center that defies the term "self-help" and acknowledges the Higher Power as essential to recovery, but I was a long way from personally experiencing that level yet.

Back at the ranch I was traversing the career path of the public-sector psychiatrist. More and more I held in awe the strength and resourcefulness of the local AA community. They were always there when they were needed, volunteering their time and concern for other drunks like themselves. They had meetings at night, at noon, on Sundays, Saturdays, in churches, furniture stores, office buildings, neighborhood houses, you name it. We could never pay for these kinds of services at the mental health center. This was all gratis, on-the-house, and from the heart. I found myself being envious of the recovering alcoholic. Not only did they seem to "have something" that I didn't, they also had each other. They believed in each other. They had credibility with each other. I felt, at best, like a kid looking through the knothole in the right-field fence without a ticket of admission and, at worst, like the bastard at a family reunion.

It was not until a decade later during the next chapter of my professional and personal career that I was able to surmount these feelings and find a more comfortable place in this alcoholic-doctor dyad. My experiences were telling me that something powerful was altering the lives of patients in the Program. I was beginning to realize that this "something powerful" was indeed a spiritual presence, this God of their understanding. I could understand that; at least I was beginning to be able to, given my own shaky state of personal spirituality.

There I went and said the "S" word again. Most people think that psychiatrists are atheists, right? After all, Freud was an atheist, so all psychiatrists must be. Psychiatrists say God is only a fantasized, institutionalized father figure, and religion is for guilt-ridden people, right? Wrong. Some of those postulates were (and are) founded in psychoanalytic theses. Even though they have now passed their heyday, I had been swept up in that scene and, for twenty of my middle years, I had been essentially an agnostic.

Some elaboration on my story is necessary at this point, to clarify the confusion that was my personal spiritual state when I met Dale.

To begin this part of the story, let me say that my mother is the soul of patience. She may have anguished privately over the fallen state of my spiritual life, but outwardly she maintained a serene confidence that "Bill will come back one day." That oft-heard refrain of hers capsuled the journey I was making, a journey I couldn't encompass in my own visual field, but one that her faith allowed her to see clearly.

She had raised me *right*. More correctly, I should say that she and my father did. I focus on her, though, because she represents, in my mind, the carrier of the faith in her generation. Hers was a replicated role of her own mother, my Grandmother Englebert, who was looked upon as the standard-bearer of her generation. My father and grandfather were church-going, God-fearing people also, but they did not radiate the faith as did the women.

"The Faith" in our family was Methodism. It was not the high-church Methodism that clings to Anglicanism in an ambivalent rebellion. This was Methodism that was imbued with the same sort of rural South fervor that today energizes the fundamentalist revival. My first church, Epworth Methodist, was a small cotton-mill-village church that rang of good old hymns, like "Bringing in the Sheaves" and "In the Sweet Bye-and-Bye." My father would sometimes lead the singing with his mellow but untrained baritone. There would be a call to the altar at the end of the service, for anyone heretofore unsaved, to answer the call to Christ and join the church.

The highlight of the church year, though, was Easter Sunday. Not because of crowded pews, brilliant spring outfits, or anticipation of the words to the final triumphant hymn, "He arose, He arose, Hallelujah, Christ arose." No, the real anticipation was the annual spirit-filling of one of the elderly women of the church. Each Easter, like clockwork, this particular gray-haired matron would pass into a trance-like state, complete with shouts and faints and much commotion, that usually ended with her being gently carried out so the service could continue. I recall sitting on the pew with my sister and cousin, whispering our anxious delights to each other, listening for the first telltale sounds from the direction of the row where she sat, sounds that signaled the warming-up that would soon lead to a full-fledged visitation of the Spirit. There was as much embarrassment, I believe, among the congregation as there was rejoicing about her episodes — which perhaps revealed the lingering Anglican/Methodist strains that did not harmonize so well with such charismatic outbursts.

No doubt about it: I was reared in what would be called a fundamentalist environment, but it was not oppressively so. Hellfire and damnation, though we may have encountered them on Sundays, were not preached at home. Also, the situation was moderated when our family changed its membership to First Methodist Church down-town, sometime around my junior high school years. The handsome building, large choir and pipe organ, and upscale trappings all mitigated any inclinations toward glossolalia among the members. Easter from then on was not nearly as exciting, but my religious education, nourished in a somewhat more enlightened environment, was the beneficiary of this change of scenery.

It never occurred to me, that I recall, to doubt anything I was taught about God or the Bible during those years at home.

Something happened, though, when I left the comfortable neigh-borhood that was Huntsville, Alabama, and ventured to Vanderbilt University in Nashville. It was only a two-and-one-half hour trip up the highway, but it might as well have been another country or era, in terms of the difference in culture.

An anecdote from my freshman year may help to symbolize something of the culture shock I experienced as a small-town Alabama collegian. I was on choir tour with the Vanderbilt A Cappella Choir that year. We were in Birmingham, and another tenor and I were being treated to a fine seated dinner in the Mountainbrook home of some very gracious hosts. Iced tea was served, and I couldn't spot the sugar bowl. Instead, I noticed these small glass, Munchkin-sized bowls at each place with a white crystalline substance in them, accompanied by a tiny spoon. As I began to tediously spoon the "sugar" into my glass of tea, milligram at a time, the lady of the house cleared her throat and politely asked, "Bill, do you always use salt in your tea?"

Just as my dinner table customs were being overhauled, so was my world view. It was in the second semester of my freshman year, approximately January of 1954. The course was "History of Western Philosophy" and was taught by a professor who could have been right out of Dickens. His clothes always looked slept in, and day-old chalk clung to his longish fingernails. He had a habit of never looking directly at us in class, but he cast his eyes upward as he mumbled dates and names and ideas, as if he were reading them from cue cards on the ceiling.

Nevertheless, teach us he did, and I was flooded with astounding revelations. WOW!! *Aristotle* wasn't a *Christian*?? (Maybe I had never bothered previously to match up the centuries; if anything happened before 1492, it was all of one piece to me.) Prior to this, I thought that arguments in theology had to do only with Yahweh *versus* God the Trinity. It never occurred to me that serious-minded people – I suppose Locke, Hume, and Nietzche fill that bill – would need to *prove* the deity's existence. It was awesome.

If Western Philosophy was "Mind-Blowing 101," then Embryology had to be 301. This was my third year in college, just prior to my entrance to medical school. Embryology was the one course that was to convince me of the beauty and truth of evolutionary theory. We studied in minute detail the progressive development of the chick embryo. We saw it pass through stages where it was practically indistinguishable from a fish embryo. Then the "gills" gave way to lungs, as the grotesque-appearing organism worked its way up the evolutionary scale. Here was BY-GOD-PROOF of evolution right before my microscope-assisted eyes.

I remember being so excited about the "find" that I wanted to announce it to anyone who would listen. I didn't realize that this had already been tried once in Tennessee, not too many miles away from Nashville, by a teacher named Scopes. Being no crusader, though, I didn't attract as much attention as he did. I just studied hard and let the new stuff wash over me. The shibboleth "Ontogeny recapitulates philogeny" stuck in my mind equally as strongly as "In the beginning God . . ." The contradictions between creationist ideology and evolution were so obvious to me that one of them had to go; and by this time in my scientific development, there was no contest.

Hindsight allows me to see that I was angry at this point. I felt betrayed, believing that I had been handed a pack of lies by my church, the Bible, even my family. Couple this with a growing sense of power that I felt with the humanistic sciences at my disposal, and I had all the makings of an avowed agnostic.

Peer relationships did nothing to stem the tide, as fellow medical students and psychiatry residents seemed to be drifting with the same current. I honestly do not recall a single classroom encounter with students or professors, once I was into medical school, in which religion was the prime topic of conversation. There was one close friend, also to become a psychiatrist, with whom I did some fairly deep soul-searching, but mostly we had intellectual discussions about theological matters.

My medical school days saw me giving little time to organized religion. My wife, Elise, kept up connections with Belmont and McKendree Methodist churches in Nashville, and I accompanied her for perfunctory appearances on occasion. We had married in 1956, the summer after I had completed undergraduate school, the chick embryo fresh in my mind's eye. Sometime in my third year of medical school, our own embryo implanted, and the Goodson family was on the way. By the end of my intern year, Dorothy and Cindy were accompanying their mother to Sunday school classes, while Dad was putting in long hours in a short white coat.

It was something of a coincidence that my psychiatric residency in 1961 took us to Belmont, Massachusetts, hotbed of Unitarianism. The Worldwide Secretary of the Unitarian Universalist Church lived just up Mill Street from us. I recall his telling of his success in recruiting no less than Albert Schweitzer into membership, simply by writing him a letter and inviting him. Schweitzer allegedly wrote back, "I'd love to; no one ever asked before." Well, now, if it was good enough for Al, it surely was good enough for me. So Elise and I made a few forays into the Belmont Unitarian Church on Sundays, taking our two daughters for what passed as Sunday School. We never made very good Unitarians, however, finding the people friendly and inviting but the services relatively unrewarding and sterile. This compromise with my mother and John Wesley wasn't going to work.

Such was my state of affairs as I was encountering alcoholism in the emergency room/bus ticket office in 1964. And such it was, more or less, for the next fifteen years of my life. A two-year tour as Division Psychiatrist with the 82nd Airborne did nothing to touch a spiritual nerve; except, perhaps, when I was about to exit the jump door of a C-131 for the first time at sixteen hundred feet with a drill sergeant's foot in my back. I think I may have murmured something theological, like, "Oh my God! Why am I doing this?" Likewise, my challenging and busy career at the Huntsville-Madison County Mental Health Center in the seventies didn't allow me the time or energy, so I thought, to pursue personal religion.

On reflection, it may have been no accident that the major model of psychological intervention at our mental health center was behavior modification. B. F. Skinner, the founding father of behaviorism, was never the favorite of the clergy. Indeed, choosing this model probably mirrored my own failure to acknowledge the need in therapeutic matters for spirituality to be regarded as a prime ingredient of *la condition humaine*.

By 1978 I had run out my string. Things had turned sour for me at the mental health center. I couldn't recognize it at the time, but my failure there was directly proportional to the ego-involvement I had with the job; i.e., the feeling that I personally was responsible for making it work. Such a conclusion is pure folly, of course, in a system as complex as a large community mental health center; but I couldn't see that.

It was this crisis in my life — my own personal "bottom" — that became a major turning point. It was about this time that I began to doubt the agnostic posture I had espoused with such confidence for so long. I looked around me and saw dozens of people I admired and respected who were in church on Sundays and on their knees at night. My poignant failures had led me to desire a knowledge of something beyond myself.

My mother's simple words were echoing: "Bill will come back one day." She seemed to have learned her text well, as in Deuteronomy 4:9: "Only take heed to thyself, and keep thy soul diligently, lest thou forget the things which thine eyes have seen, and lest they depart from thy heart all the days of thy life; but teach them thy sons, and thy sons' sons."

Important to my story and Dale's is the fact that I had come to the point when I was ready to revisit the notion that God is at work in our lives. This allowed some other things to happen; namely, the door was open for me to begin to understand what was happening to my alcoholic patients in recovery, and for the first time, my encounters with them had a chance of being mutually enriching.

God *was* at work in 1979. Some thought maybe the office upstairs had been vacated during the Iranian hostage crisis, but I have rather convincing evidence otherwise. You might call it serendipity, or synchronicity, or coincidence; but an opportunity came my way. As I was exiting the public-sector mental health field and entering private practice again, there was at the same time a small psychiatric unit at Crestwood Hospital about to be closed. The psychiatrist who had kept the program alive was moving out. Taking a leaf from nature's book, I moved into the vacuum and saw a chance to establish the first chemical dependency unit in Huntsville. I thought we needed one, and others confirmed that. Before making any commitments, however, I talked it over with Bob R., who by then also had left community mental health work. He, too, thought it a good idea. I told him I would do it only if he would agree to work in the unit. He did, and I did, and we did.

A year later in 1980, Dale was admitted to the Crestwood A & D Unit. I had a year under my belt as Medical Director of the treatment unit. We had assembled a competent staff, with a blend of recovering and nonrecovering persons. As with all such programs of that day, we leaned heavily on the AA and NA programs for program content and direction. The psychiatric staff (there were only two of us) handled the medical aspects of detoxification and other physical aspects of treatment and also directed the psychological aspects of patient care. But with most patients, after the initial phases, I found I had little to offer in the way of psychiatric or medical expertise.

In fact, by the time Dale was admitted, I was beginning to wonder if a psychiatrist was very useful in an alcohol treatment center. My understandings had led me to this critical point of doubt. I knew that much of what I did with these patients in the hospital could be done by an internist or family practitioner trained in addiction medicine. A cascade of research in the sixties and seventies had demonstrated conclusively that psychotherapy and psychotropic drugs were not the answer for the average alcoholic. So if I couldn't analyze or drug them out of their inebriation, what *could* I do?

I could get out of the way, for one thing. What with everyone getting their "by-pass" these days, I could engage in psychiatric by-pass therapy. By-pass the psychiatrist. Get on to the recovery program. Don't get bogged down in exploring the psyche, the attachment to mother, dependency issues, etc. And for God's sake, don't offer a chemical solution (medications) to the person who is chemically dependent. Talk about fanning the fire. Get out of the way and let the Program do its work. Then comes the obvious question: Why a psychiatrist at all? What is the use of psychiatric expertise in the treatment of the chemically dependent person?

Given this level professional nihilism and mortification, you might be expecting me to terminate my portion of the book at this point and leave the rest for Dale to tell his story. The book outline would then go something like this:

Dr. Goodson meets Dale.

Dr. Goodson gets out of the way.

Dale recovers.

But, I did not exit the scene. My own journey was unfolding, as was Dale's. I was just a few years ahead of Dale in reaching my nadir of personal despair. Clearly, though, we were in this thing together.

CHAPTER

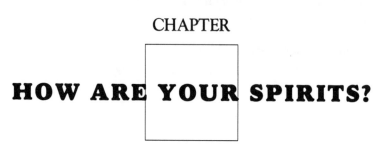

HOW ARE YOUR SPIRITS?

T H R E E

"How are your spirits today, Dale?" A typical question I might ask him during his hospital stay, but a question with a hidden agenda. If you are looking for triple entendres, you can find one here. This question could be interpreted very concretely as, "How is your liquor supply?" The "spirits" could also refer to the soul, the spirit, the spiritual seat of the person. Most commonly, of course, it is an inquiry about mood. On the surface the alcoholic's problem is the liquor cabinet. But the psyche and the soul are the deeper problems that need attention in recovery.

Dale was depressed, no doubt about it. Alcohol was controlling his life in spite of his promises to his wife, doctor, God; in spite of his progressive loss of effectiveness on his job as an FBI agent; in spite of his diminished life at home and in the community. Plenty to be depressed about. His second round of treatment in as many months. How did his life get in such a mess? As Henry said to Eleanor in *The Lion in Winter*, "step by step."

Two major eras marked Dale's life until that time. They could be called "Life Without Booze" and "Life With Booze." As befitted a product of the fifties, Dale wasn't into drinking in his early years. A couple of debauches in high school and college was about all there was to it. Dale married early, spent four years in the Air Force, then finished college. Goal-directedness claimed him, leaving little time for fun and games — or drinking. He was drunk only twice while in the service. A brief stint teaching high school math in California taught him he wanted a graduate degree, which he promptly attained. He simply wasn't exposed to much drinking during those years; maybe a punch bowl at a wedding, but he usually chose cake and coffee.

The second era in Dale's life was heralded by his decision to quit teaching and join the FBI. This brought about changes not only in his work but also in the lifestyle and friendships he cultivated. With his professional career came a thriving, middle-class life, including church, school, and social activities. And with financial security came a new range of activities with a common "wet" texture: activities such as bridge, poker, Quarterback Club, Elks Club, Officer's Club, and ball games. As their children grew older (he and Mary Lou had three), there was more free time for dining, dancing, and nightclubs. Dale found himself in front of a tidal wave of ethanol, but not necessarily a menacing one. This was a tidal wave disguised as a hot tub. Dale found inebriation to be soothing and pleasant.

In a very different way from his adolescent and military experience with alcohol — which were isolated, impulsive, and ultimately unpleasant — Dale now experienced the euphoric and disinhibiting effects of ethyl alcohol in a gentler, kinder environment. He was consorting with mature, successful, respected members of his community, and he was one of them. They all drank — well, ninety percent did — and drank regularly. Whatever insecurities and anxieties he may have brought with him to social encounters were dissipated with the lubrication of drink.

With this classic seduction came the inevitable progression of the illness. Wait a minute! Hold the phone! Illness? Who said anything about an illness? Most certainly Dale did not *feel* sick. He felt good. He felt so good that soon he was drinking when there were no social reasons. First, a drink on weekends; then, buying and keeping liquor in his home. The erosion of control was so gradual hardly anyone noticed. From 1968 to 1972 he had matured into a five-day-a-week pint drinker. The progression was logical: It's okay to have a few indulgences on the weekend, right? Saturday is the herald-day; Fridays are weekends, too. It doesn't take much imagination to see that Thursdays are *really* preambles to the weekends, and Sundays should not be excluded from the number. Stretching things a bit allows Wednesday to nestle into the fold. And that pretty much completes the outline for a five-day binge.

By 1974, Dale was drinking a pint daily, seven days a week. No longer did he pressure himself to rationalize his habit. He didn't try to justify to himself what he was doing. He was simply addicted to the use of alcohol. Not that he was experiencing withdrawal symptoms (the shakes, or DTs); that would come later. But he was no longer in control of his drinking. What had begun with innocent social drinking was, by then, a compulsive habit. His brain and his psyche were so accustomed to the enhancing effects of ethanol that he was dependent upon it.

It took four more years for his required intake to escalate to a fifth daily. By 1978 his life was revolving around alcohol consumption. When company would leave after an evening at his home, he would clean up the alcohol as well as the house. At BYOB parties he would steal from others to keep his supply intact. He always volunteered to tend bar, at home or away, to stay close to the action and assure his supply. All social events deteriorated to those where alcohol was available. Often this meant sneaking it into ball games, movies, or even a child's birthday party!

Fear began to creep in as he saw his control over his life erode. Most of all, however, he was preoccupied with the fear of losing his job.

Dale had served most of his twenty years with the Bureau under the scrutiny of J. Edgar Hoover, whose primary management philosophy was "rule by fear" — which meant perfection and an absolute certainty of swift punishment. Voluminous policy manuals covered every known possible infraction relating to the job or personal life. Policy violations usually meant dismissal without appeal.

Dale initially loved his work, even under the tyrannical administration, because it was rewarding, and the system fostered success. He progressed through his career at an above-average pace and was exemplary. Unknown to all (even Dale), he was toting the baggage of alcoholism up his career ladder. Toward the end of his days with the FBI, his disease had begun to progress faster than Dale. It was way ahead of him when, in 1978, he was appointed head of his own FBI office, with more than a dozen agents working with and for him. By that time he had already lost complete control to alcohol.

Prior to his promotion, Dale had managed to escape detection quite well by being a loner, working long hours away from the office (and from Mary Lou) to avoid associating with people. That made it less likely someone could smell his always-laden breath. He could work from his car by radio, talk with informants, use a telephone, keep a safe distance from people with cough drops on his breath, and deal with people who didn't care. He was a good report writer and produced statistics that were impressive.

Believing he could control his drinking, Dale accepted the promotion because it would be financially rewarding, then and in retirement. Retirement pay was based on last salary level; he didn't need his math major to see that meant a lot of money to him.

Little did he dream the mental hell and anguish this move would mean to him. Right from the start of his new assignment, Dale was drinking every day. The first year he managed to maintain a long morning of productive work to keep everything looking good. He would then leave in mid-afternoon, "going to a meeting," and, on the rare occasion he needed to return, he would wait until evening when the office was empty.

There were some aspects of the situation that were ideal for an alcoholic. For one thing, Dale was in charge and answered only to the state director, a hundred miles away. The director visited only once or twice a year, and then by appointment made long in advance. (Dale could still abstain for a few hours at those times.) Additionally, none of his employees could confront him since he did their performance evaluations and recommended their promotions and awards. Dale knew if they looked good, he looked good, so he recommended everyone as often as possible for promotion. Things were nice and tidy.

Fear, however, would not leave him alone. A couple of years after his promotion, Dale became very concerned that someone would realize he was drinking on duty every day and report him. He was well aware of FBI policy and knew that employees had been dismissed for lesser offenses. Dwelling on this thought soon magnified it to an obsession. He realized retirement was just two years away, and if he were fired for drinking, he would lose everything he had worked for − not only his reputation but also a small fortune. He had calculated that if he lived to an age of seventy years, he would draw retirement payments of almost half a million dollars; and if dismissed in his nineteenth year of service, he would get nothing!

He read the FBI policy manual until it was ingrained in his memory: On the very first page, second only to "employees must not engage in criminal or immoral conduct," he read, "Agents should never cause themselves to be mentally or physically unfit on duty, so the use of alcoholic beverages is not permitted during working hours, including any time allotted for meal periods or any period of annual leave taken if the agent returns to work before the end of the working day." Any doubt that he would be dismissed if found drinking on duty was removed when Dale noted that alcohol abuse was listed *ahead* of other serious-sounding restrictions, such as, "FBI agents shall not accept rewards or gratuities, engage in entrapment, purloin or misuse government property, or join the Communist Party." Convinced that he could not stop drinking and that his entire future depended on his retirement, he lived with a twenty-four-hour-a-day obsession to hide his drinking at work. He became paranoid around his co-workers. Hall's Mentholyptus was not the panacea he had hoped!

Whenever Dale had a duty that could not be ignored, canceled, delayed, or handled by a subordinate, by letter, or by telephone, he would be forced to schedule a personal appointment in his office. Early on he had rearranged his office with an oversized desk between him and all visitors' chairs, which were located as far away as possible. Thus, with windows open and a mouthful of cough drops, it was hard to smell the faint vodka breath. He even gave thought to starting to smoke again, maybe even cigars!

As time went on, Dale's fears began to overwhelm him. He realized he could not continue his charade, and he initiated a geographic cure.

In 1980 he requested — and was overjoyed when he was granted — a demotion and was assigned to work alone in two rural Alabama counties. Alone, with no one to answer to, he was again in a position to devote much time to his dipsomania.

The predictable result occurred. Dale was hospitalized for detoxification four times by his family physician and attended two separate alcohol and drug treatment centers (Atlanta and Crestwood — the episodes described in Chapter One) in the last two years of his government service, 1980 to 1982. His accompanying decline in health and character was obvious to everyone, yet Dale absurdly demanded to stay in control of his life on his own terms, vehemently denying that alcohol was his master.

The last few months before his retirement were lived in an alcoholic fog where the absolute minimum was accomplished, and Dale visited his office only when he had to. His greatest achievement of this period was getting his paycheck in the bank by direct deposit so he wouldn't even have to appear on payday.

"How are your spirits?" Dale's were moving toward an all-time low. There was no joy in his life. He was the dog chasing its tail and pacing himself one step ahead of the shakes. A treadmill is no fun, particularly when the end isn't in sight, and Dale was looking downward all the time just to keep his balance. Whereas alcohol used to facilitate interaction and elevate his mood, at this point it was scarcely sufficient to keep him from feeling miserable. He was able to gather himself together enough to go through the motions, but barely so. Things were going badly at home as well. Mary Lou's attitude had vacillated from despair to anger to pity, and everyone close to Dale felt helpless. He had "become" an alcoholic through a long metamorphosis that was so slow, subtle, and beguiling that it went virtually undetected until the demon was in absolute control of his mind, body, and spirit.

As if this scenario weren't depressing enough, Dale was also suffering an accumulating load of grief from his losses during the previous decade. By the end of the 1970s, he was the sole survivor in his family of origin. In 1972 alone, he unexpectedly lost his brother-in-law (with whom he had been very close), his father-in-law, and his own beloved mother. Mary Lou's mother died in 1970. Add to that the death of his brother's wife's in 1976, and his own father, the venerable patriarch, in 1978. Wasn't that enough?

Not quite. I left out the one that hurt the most: Dale's only brother, Curtis, died suddenly in 1975. Curtis was easily Dale's best friend. He was also a mentor and confidant. And he was alcoholic. Curtis killed himself. No one talked about it much, and for years Dale himself tried to deny the truth of it, fabricating some theory of foul play. But the truth is that Curtis was alcoholic, and he committed suicide, throwing himself from a building in Chicago.

Dale carried a burden of guilt about his brother's death for a long time. He recalls it this way:

> *During the two months before Curtis died – that was in 1975 – I got three emergency phone calls from Chicago, from this friend of his who was a priest. Curtis was drinking, so he was in bad need of help. The first time, I dropped everything and went up to Chicago to help him dry out – the blind leading the blind.*
>
> *Of course, Curtis promised to stay sober and all that.*

*The second time, I flew there again, and his friend
and I tried to get Curtis admitted to a treatment center
north of Chicago. Curtis backed out on the doorstep.*

*The third time was too much. I told his friend I wasn't
coming up there again. It just wasn't doing any good.
Two weeks afterward, I got another call with the news
that Curtis was dead.*

For each of the family member's funerals, Dale and Mary Lou flew
back to their home state of Minnesota. It seemed they were the only
members of the clan to leave the Gopher state, so the Huntsville-
Minneapolis flyway was busy. Dale managed to keep the flight attendants busy, too, refilling his glass. He medicated his way through those
funerals, recalling little about whom he shook hands with and staggering
a great deal. He was particularly drunk ("obnoxiously disrespectful," as
Mary Lou described him) at his father's funeral, having downed a quart
of vodka just prior to the service. He had to be helped down the aisle
to the family pew by two ushers. Dale vaguely recalls whispered
comments such as, "Dale sure is taking it hard"; "Dale sure is worn out;
he came a long way"; "Dale looks drunk — but he couldn't be — he's
in charge of a big FBI office in Alabama."

Dale had no chance to resolve his grief. Alcohol numbed him to
his feelings, keeping them well hidden and suppressed. It was only much
later in treatment that he was to dig down and find the pocket of grief
he had walled off and had been adding to his depression.

On top of all this, Dale's relationships with his three children were
suffering, much more than he realized at the time. It was impossible for
them to get through to him, through the fog of his illness, to commu-

nicate their true feelings. When they eventually were able to express their feelings in writing, their pain, as it mirrored Dale's, became evident:

From Brad: "*I have seen you go from a very proud FBI agent to a depressed retired person. . . . When sober, you are much easier to get close to, you are loving and friendly. When you are drunk, you become loud, bullheaded, and very mean. . . . I have seen you abuse Mom verbally and emotionally . . .*"

From Deb: "*I could see you living your life in an alcoholic fog . . . always with a drink in your hand. You couldn't seem to enjoy life without it. . . . I sometimes felt compassion or pity to see you ruining your life. . . . I felt hurt because you seemed so far away . . . so removed . . . as if you didn't love us anymore.*"

And finally, from Jeff: "*I see your drinking robbing you of happiness. It changes you so dramatically. I know it's killing you . . . but still the love is there. I love you! I cry about our lives, but they're not over yet . . .*"

Clearly, family relationships were damaged. Mary Lou was very much aware of these tortured feelings and did her best to keep hope alive. Many of the children's comments reflected that ray of hope, as well as the losses, they were feeling about their dad's drinking. Dale was losing his children and was only half-consciously aware of it.

Perhaps Dale's most telling loss of this decade, however, was his loss of the ability to choose *not* to drink, the ability to drink like normal people. But he continued to delude himself. He was absolutely convinced, without a shred of doubt, that "somehow, someday he would control and enjoy his drinking." A few years later Dale saw this quotation in the book *Alcoholics Anonymous* and knew that these few simple words described his incredibly complex mental state. His fear and delusion mounted, and he spiraled downward into the echoing conclusion, "Another drink will fix it." That always seemed to be the answer: a toxic solution to survival. The ultimate oxymoron.

"How are your spirits, Dale?" He often thought of suicide during those times.

There were times when God was dead for Dale. If God couldn't pull his brother, Curtis, through; if God could let Curtis kill himself, then what could God possibly do for Dale? Curtis, the Lutheran theologian, the first Protestant to teach on the faculty of the Roman Catholic school of theology at DePaul University. Curtis, recognized by Mayor Daley of Chicago for his ecumenical work in the city. Curtis, who was knighted by the King of Sweden in 1966 for his scholarly work and who published no less than seven books to the glory of God. It was this Curtis that the God of Dale's religious understanding had abandoned.

Lest we blame Dale's spiritual decline altogether on this one event, however, it is well to note that Dale's religious life — not unlike mine — had been in a state of decline for many years. We both had allowed this to happen as we drifted through the past two decades, the major difference being that I didn't have a single, dramatic event around which to mobilize my anger toward God, as Dale did.

Dale had been reared in a strict conservative Lutheran church and had been the model church-going youngster, a leader of his youth group, a Boy Scout, a choir member, and an acolyte. His experience matched very closely my own Methodist version, where I had been president of the Methodist Youth Fellowship and a choir member, as a teen-ager.

He had been encouraged by his family to follow in Curtis' footsteps and study for the ministry. But Dale's interests lay elsewhere, and he pursued a teaching degree in math and science. By the time he was married with children, he had long lost any semblance of religious stirrings and was keeping up the ingrained practice of church life primarily in an attempt to raise his children properly.

He knew he was being hypocritical. He was troubled and confused, still nurturing doubts that had accumulated since childhood — doubts about the church of his misunderstanding. He continued to believe in God, but he found it hard to live with his lack of complete understanding.

During this span of years, he had turned frequently to Curtis for guidance. Dale and his brother had numerous, lengthy, soul-searching discussions. It was comforting to Dale that his theologically-learned mentor also had been perplexed sometimes. They had shared correspondence, and Curtis's writings often had been pithy. Of the many writings from Curtis' letters that Dale has kept and shared with others, there is one that seems to have foreshadowed Dale's eventual recovery through AA: "*No person can exist in total isolation from God and fellowman. For the Christian understanding is that no one is ever alone but always lives and grows in community, in fellowship with others.*"

It was a doubly cruel irony that, as the years went by, Dale and Curtis's late-into-the-night discussions became more and more accompanied by drinking; and that Curtis never experienced the "living and growing" of an AA community.

Despite Dale's bursts of questing and church activity, his inner spirits continued to flag as his alcoholism progressed. By 1975, when he no longer felt compelled to put up a religious front for the children (they were in college or beyond), he severed ties with the church and drifted further and further away from a relationship with God. He developed a Job-complex, what with all the deaths in the family (especially Curtis'), his home being destroyed by a tornado, and his own failing physical, mental, and spiritual health. All the remorse, guilt, grief, and anger were neutralized by alcohol, as was his quest for God.

So the question "How are your spirits" was a tough one for Dale. He flunked the quiz in all three areas: alcohol, soul, and mood. He had many reasons to be depressed: threatened loss of job, potential estrangement from his wife, distancing of his children, and high blood pressure.

His family physician had been astute in suspecting Dale's depression to be a problem in and of itself. By the time I came into the picture, the exact nature of Dale's problems were still not clear; i.e., whether depression was altogether related to grief and despair, or whether he had a mood disorder independent of alcohol. It was not until later, after several episodes of treatment with him, that his clinical features began to materialize more clearly out of the fog. It was then up to me to refine the diagnosis and orchestrate the treatment.

Voila! I *do* have a legitimate place in treating the alcoholic. I'm not relegated to the realm of "bypass" psychiatry. Indeed, I can be like an orchestra conductor. When there are complex issues, and there often are, my job is to beat time and summon the sections as needed to round out the performance. My career went from bus ticket agent to symphonic conductor, in the wink of a bloodshot eye.

Why was this important for me? What difference did it make that I found a niche in this sector of clinical work? I could have directed a career toward any of a number of different areas: adult psychotherapy, geriatrics, adolescents, forensics, to name a few. Had the treatment of alcoholics lost its appeal to me, I may have done so. Had the management of chemical dependence not challenged me to use all the tools acquired in medical school, residency, and practice, I may have drifted away in search of more satisfying pastures. The reality was, though, that I did find many satisfactions working with patients in recovery. My motivations were complex and rooted in my own personal history — in my spiritual journey and in other dimensions of my life.

The Dales and Bobs I encountered were surrounding me with their lives — lives of despair mixed with hope. Dale seemed to be on a path of inevitable self-destruction. Much of his grief, he was not sharing with me — or with anyone, for that matter. He kept me on the surface of his life, which irritated me because it was a reminder to me of his failure to comes to terms with his problem.

Early in his treatment I couldn't foresee that his course would be so involved and challenging. I never knew which patients — especially alcoholics — would stick with treatment or disappear from sight. I had learned not to let my ego get too involved in their recovery. So I kept an emotional distance from Dale; even though I liked him, I didn't want to let my desire for his recovery outmatch his. That was one of the lessons Bob R. taught me: "You're in trouble when *you* want the drunks to get sober more than *they* do." I haven't always been able to adhere to those words of wisdom, but I was getting better at it by the time Dale came along.

I was learning to *hang in there* without getting *hung up*.

I was hanging in there with Dale and others; and they were hanging in there with me.

CHAPTER

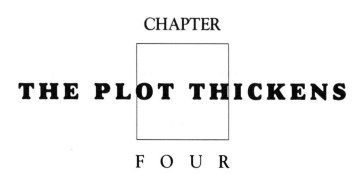

THE PLOT THICKENS

F O U R

"God, this is Bill Goodson. Grant me the patience to be patient with my patients..." So would go my Serenity Prayer, especially in dealings with alcoholics. Such was my prayer — long and often — with Dale over the next few years. There would be numerous opportunities to give up on him: when he canceled appointments, refused to be hospitalized, blatantly planned drinking binges, denied his need for AA. The list could go on. He would drop out of sight for months on end — the tell-tale sign of another drinking episode. Then suddenly he would appear again in one of several familiar scenarios: back in the hospital for drying out; or on my appointment schedule (urgent, of course), returning sheepishly to report his unruly behavior; or desperately depressed and suicidal, ready to be hospitalized.

Somehow Dale had made it to retirement in 1982 — by the grace of God and the skin of his teeth. Being of a restless nature, however, he was soon looking for other employment. His old profession, teaching, beckoned, and he took and passed the state exam for teachers. You might ask, "How does a fifty-year-old drunk who has mercilessly slaughtered his brain cells for years pass a teachers' exam?" The answer is twofold: He still had a generous supply of remaining gray matter, and he could at times summon up enough control over his drinking (with the help of Antabuse) to function adequately for short periods of time. So Dale was preparing to teach high school or college math and, in the meantime, to occupy himself with part-time substitute teaching in the city school system.

His new career was marred with a few interruptions. Twice in a two-month span in 1983, Dale was so disturbed that he needed intensive treatment, not in the Crestwood Unit but in a "real" psychiatric unit at Huntsville Hospital, the city-county general hospital. The first such admission followed a very bizarre episode. So bizarre, in fact, that it defied explanation as a product of his drinking.

A somewhat different picture was beginning to emerge, indicating that Dale was experiencing a psychotic depression, a depression so profound that he had lost touch with reality. Perhaps this is most vividly demonstrated by my notes from that hospital admission:

"About two weeks ago when I saw Dale in the office, he related to me an unusual incident in which he had awakened, felt that he had some particular mission to perform, and was in something of a dream-like state.... I was unsure whether ... he was entering a psychotic state.... He told me that in the last week or so he had developed mental confusion, doubts about his own mental capacities. The other day, when he was substitute teaching at Huntsville High School, he was unable to do a simple arithmetic problem on the board, became distraught about this ... later went home, was watching the Donohue show. It had to do with the new mayor of Chicago, and Dale became quite involved in the implications of this, thinking about the social problems of the world and where it was all headed. He became very morbid and pessimistic."

Never before had Dale reached such a point, though there had been signs of significant depression. In fact, a year prior to this, a cyclic nature in his moods had appeared. Mary Lou and his children noted an approximate six-week duration of these cycles in which he would be unusually cheerful and active for a while, followed by weeks of inactivity and poor spirits. This description, coupled with my own observations, had led me to suggest he have another try at taking lithium carbonate, the treatment of choice for manic depression or Bipolar Disorder. I was ninety percent sure, at this point, that his chromosomes harbored a "blues gene." Unfortunately, Dale didn't stay sober long enough to assess the impact of the medication. He didn't stay sober long enough for much of anything in those days.

The presence of the second psychiatric disorder in Dale was confusing to all concerned: himself, Mary Lou, and his medical helpers. His chemical dependency counselors (and probably the AA members he had encountered) had seen in him what they had come to expect as depression in the recovering alcoholic. Depression often appears, as it did with Dale, related variously to guilt, discouragement (as with relapses), PLOMS (Poor Little Old Me Syndrome), persistent craving for a drink, and a host of other recovery issues. Dale's mood disorder had roots in the alcoholic realm, as well as in his genes.

He was in good company. This scenario is familiar to those knowledgable about AA history. The founder of AA, Bill Wilson, fought depression for a decade or more, many years after his last drink. He sought relief through the Program; he consulted psychiatrists; he took LSD and vitamins. According to his biographers (in *Pass It On*), he was often advised by friends that he wasn't working his Program properly, etc. Had he been fast-forwarded twenty years, he probably would have found relief much sooner than he did, with the use of antidepressants. As it was, he had to struggle through those perplexing times, as did Dale and I.

Working with the diagnosis of psychotic depression, I prescribed an antidepressant and antipsychotic drugs. Dale's thinking cleared and his depression began to lift. He stayed on the psychiatric unit at Huntsville a total of fifteen days, a relatively brief time considering the severity of his condition on admission. It seemed that Dale might be out of the woods; maybe we had found the answer. He was discharged taking his new medications, and Antabuse, and with an understanding he would not try to work right away.

Unaccustomed to following others' advice, Dale immediately accepted a position teaching criminal justice during summer session at a local university. Bizarre things began to happen again. He gave his students an exam that didn't make sense and then resigned his position. He embarked on a stock-trading spree that cost him several thousand dollars. Within a month, Mary Lou called in a panic, and we agreed that Dale belonged back in the hospital. He checked in and then signed out a day later. After much cajoling, he finally agreed to come in and stay. This time he was in a confused state of mind and with suicidal ideation.

At this point the diagnosis was one hundred percent clear. Dale's manic buying spree was the final tip-off, the absolute clincher — this was indeed a Bipolar Disorder. Dale would have to take lithium for an extended time in order to control his moods. Of course, I had suspected this earlier, but perhaps I hadn't been convinced enough of the diagnosis to push hard for sustained lithium therapy — and the fact that Dale did not stay sober would have made it impossible to discern the efficacy of the medications anyway.

Dale then proceeded to have his best year in a long time. He didn't drink, kept his appointments with me, took lithium, and taught courses at various local institutions. The lithium had some side effects (mainly tremors and coordination problems), but he managed to tolerate them, and his moods were much improved. Mary Lou was happier, too. She was ensuring her mate's sobriety by watching him swallow an Antabuse tablet daily. This was a ritual that I had reluctantly condoned. Relying on Antabuse alone in treating an alcoholic is like hoping a splint will mend a displaced fracture. It might happen in one out of a hundred cases, with blind luck. Putting Mary Lou in charge of administering Antabuse was like using a cardboard splint: It was a patch-up job until the orthopedic surgeon arrived; or, in our case, until Dale decided to get serious about recovering. My faith in him and Mary Lou and the grace of God told me that we needed to keep hanging on, even if we were hanging on to a cardboard splint.

This fragile arrangement lasted until the summer of 1984, when Dale's devotion to sobriety was outmatched by the lure of a Caribbean cruise. Mary Lou had been looking forward to this diversion, with the vain hope that Dale could stay sober and avoid a booze cruise. About a week prior to embarkation, Dale announced that he was not only leaving his troubles behind, but also his Antabuse. Too late to cancel and get a rebate (Dale had planned it that way), they forged ahead, and the inevitable progression ensued. After the cruise, Dale did his best to break down the trade barriers with the Soviet Union with a single-handed assault on the Vodka supplies of the world. First weekends, then week days, and within a few months, Dale's drinking was back to a record pace.

It was a little different this time, however. He kept his appointments, took his medication (lithium plus an antidepressant), taught school, and maintained some semblance of sanity in his life — at least for a while. But, alas, even the miracles of modern chemistry couldn't protect his brain from the perpetual ethanol barrage, and eventually he quit his job, became suicidally depressed, and was back on the psych unit.

This episode of depression cleared readily after he was detoxified, demonstrating again that alcohol played a significant role in his mood problems. This time around I attempted to get Dale to agree to a different sort of recovery program, suggesting long term treatment in a place such as Hazelden in Minnesota. After all, he was from Minnesota and that would be a natural, I reasoned. Dale demurred, congenially, reiterating his dislike of the AA Program and vowing to continue taking Antabuse.

Dale was still convincing himself that he could manage his drinking problem — that same old self-delusional routine he had practiced for so long.

Mary Lou was learning the basics of detachment: distancing herself emotionally and allowing Dale to take responsibility for his drinking. She immersed herself in her profession of nursing and kept hope alive with her children as best she could. She was the kind of patient's spouse psychiatrists dream of: supportive, but not intrusive.

In retrospect, it was probably Mary Lou's presence that helped to keep my hope alive for Dale. Her calm perseverance, her quiet determination to see it through, were inspirational. I can still picture her visiting on the psychiatric ward at Huntsville Hospital, patiently convincing Dale to stay there for treatment when he was in the throes of psychotic disorganization.

I think that is what we mean when we speak of "teamwork" in treating alcoholics. When I have just about given up on a patient, another of the *team* will *work* on me, by word or example, to get me to keep on.

CHAPTER

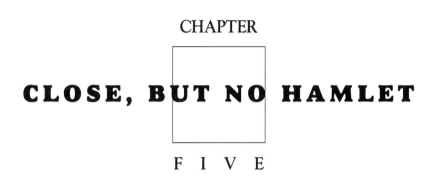

CLOSE, BUT NO HAMLET

F I V E

Trying to puzzle through Dale's illness was a real workout for me, but I had been in training for a few years, hefting around my own baggage. While I may not have been suffering from dual diagnoses, I did have two or three (at least) continuing problems to deal with – problems that directly impacted on my professional life and the particular crossroads at which I found myself. I had to find myself, professionally and spiritually. Somehow I had gotten lost.

I've already acquainted you with a bit of my youth and hometown. I mentioned a time when my family changed churches, from a small one outside the city proper to a large downtown version. That switch from Epworth Methodist to First Methodist was symbolic of a dissonant thread that has marked my life as a psychiatrist.

I'll explain that.

Huntsville in my youth (I was born there in 1936) was characterized by the stratification of society – white society, that is – along economic lines. The two poles of the cotton industry provided the demarcation: the farm and gin owners, mill officials, cotton brokers and associated money handlers at one end; and the mill workers and farm laborers at the other. The warps and the woofs of the South. The "cotton mill villages," as they were called, were just outside the city limits and so were served by the county government and a paternalistic mill ownership that provided subsidized housing, company store, YMCA, and school funding.

My father and mother, reared in that cotton mill environment, shared the mixed blessing of a fierce sense of community paired with the "other side of the tracks" syndrome. Until age five, I lived in one of those villages, called Dallas Mill Village. Then we — mother, father, sister Mary Lou (not to be confused with Dale's Mary Lou) and I — eased over into a neighborhood not far from the village, but, significantly, within the city school system.

Schools became the melting pot for Mary Lou and me, as they were for much of the community (white, that is; remember — these were the forties and fifties). Our expectations were ratcheted up several notches, as we were in daily communion with ambitions born of a vision that promised a better life. Friendships were made on the basis of innocent beliefs that we (children) were all very much the same. Since we read from the same textbooks and ate at the same tables in the school cafeteria, we didn't worry too much about socioeconomic differences. We could compete equally in the classroom and on the athletic field: Teachers awarded grades without reference to one's tax bracket, and coaches were more interested in a person's skill in passing the ball than how properly the bread was passed.

I can thank my parents for the priority given to academic pursuits in my life. Both of them came from relatively uneducated backgrounds; my paternal grandfather was only semi-literate (though he could quote much of the King James Version by heart). The sixth of seven children, my father, Houston Goodson, was destined to be the "point man" in his family, in many senses of the word, by his aggressive pursuits. Not only did he distinguish himself in athletics, but he was also the only sibling to attain a college education, one step ahead of his baby sister, Marcheta, who was high school class valedictorian. His teacher's certificate from Florence State Teachers' College marked the beginnings of a movement out of the cotton mill village, a shift that generated enough momentum to carry me along with it. Even as he became a successful businessman and prominent leader in city government as President of the City Council, my father proudly wore his up-by-the-bootstraps badge and never pretended to shed his rough-hewn ways.

Respected as he was in most quarters, it was this reputation for a rough-and-tumble style, along with some notorious episodes of immoderation with alcohol, that probably helped to spell the end of his political career. Finishing a distant third in the mayoral race of 1968, he lived out the rest of his life more privately.

He didn't do badly. The Goodsons were Scotch-Irish who came over to Virginia in the eighteenth century, along with crowds of immigrants, many of whom were probably bearing marks of a ball and chain. Mostly, they were simple working folk. One of Dad's brothers Doyle (nicknamed "Soup") was a bootlegger who had been in his share of gunfights. Uncle Soup was a man with a heart of gold and a body full of lead, a walking Periodic Table. He never would never have made it through an airport security check without prior major surgical intervention.

Though my father wasn't on the fringes of the law like his brother, he not infrequently betrayed his yeoman heritage. An anecdote from his later years will illustrate the point: He had a cabin on Guntersville Lake near Huntsville that was frequently the target of break-ins. A string of such rascally deeds had remained unimpeded by various measures, until Dad decided he had figured out who the culprit was. He then proceeded to take the law into his own hands: He went to the man's house, beat him up, called the sheriff to report what he had done (inviting the sheriff to arrest him if he wished), and went on his way. Dad was sixty-five years old at the time, the other man about forty. The break-ins ceased.

It's not difficult to understand how my father's style of conflict resolution may have tainted his public image to a degree. But this episode tells more about my Dad than just his macho disposition. It demon-strates, to be sure, his qualities of decisiveness and justice (albeit, frontier-style); but the fact that he reported his actions to the authorities also shows his honesty and respect for the law. He lived that difficult balance between individual versus corporate responsibility, between protection of self and of society, and lived it well, if not always delicately.

He left some rather large shoes to fill. I had never been able to fill them athletically, but other avenues were opening.

As my father's public life waned, mine commenced. I had become a psychiatrist and had returned to practice in my home town of Huntsville in 1966. This was hardly the cotton mill town of fifteen thousand that I had left in 1953 to begin my extramural wanderings via Vanderbilt, Boston, and the 82nd Airborne. Fifteen years and a few Sputniks later, Huntsville had been transformed into the Space Capital of the World with more Ph.D.s per capita than Route 128 in Boston. Just as my home town was different, so was I. I was imbued with the sciences of Sigmund Freud and Adolph Meyer; Huntsville, with those of Albert Einstein and Werner von Braun. I was attracted to scientific humanism; Huntsville, to humanistic science. I sported accretions of the past decade: wife, three daughters, corkscrew (I only discovered after moving to Boston that some wine bottles required such), snow skis, and a permanently disfigured Southern accent. Huntsville sported a university, German restaurants, an erstwhile bypass, and a downtown damaged at the hands of sprawling suburbs and shopping malls.

Huntsville also boasted a new vision for a mental health center. The Kennedy and Johnson administrations had midwifed the birth of the community mental health centers movement, and it was on the verge of a major growth spurt in the late 1960s. This seemed like a golden opportunity for me, one that I could not pass up.

There I was: a young psychiatrist coming back home to do something not for money (a salary of $30,000 was not high cotton, even in 1969), but to do something *significant* for my people. Maybe about ten percent of my decision was motivated by career diversity: There was a lot to be learned about community psychiatry, and this was as good a chance as any. But I suspect the other ninety percent of my move had a lot to do with me as a person, as well as a psychiatrist.

To find out more about that ninety percent, I have to ask myself a question: How did I grow up to be a psychiatrist, anyway? Why *this* specialty of medicine over all the rest? If someone had told me, when I entered medical school, that I was going into psychiatry, I would have, at the least, appeared puzzled and probably would have been amused. Psychiatry isn't the most glamorous field, it's certainly not the most lucrative, and it's often thought of as being outside the mainstream. I'm sure my father must have wondered what the heck his son was doing, spending all that time and money (mostly his) becoming a *psychiatrist*. Isn't a doctor supposed to cut and sew, take X-Rays, or at least put somebody to sleep! But talking with people and working on their minds

— that doesn't sound like a *real* man's work!

How do I know my Dad thought that? I don't, really. He was always openly supportive and generous when it came to my educational pursuits. I *imagine* he thought those things because I thought them myself, many times, for many years. Sometimes my well-thought-out career motives — to wit, being attracted to a specialty that allowed me to approach the patient from many points of view — were beset with doubts. Here I was, a mill-village boy at heart; son of a tough, fist-slinging, boot-strapping, hard-drinking, athletic, Scotch-Irish descendant; nephew of the town's most notorious bootlegger. How did I choose a "soft" field like psychiatry?

It must have been my mother. (Isn't that what we psychiatrists always say?) I never was very tough. I'd been in only one fist-fight my whole life, and that had been with my best friend in junior high school. I hadn't played high school football because I never liked the violence to my body. My mind had been ahead of my body when I walked to the stage on Awards Day. Even at my best sport, basketball, I couldn't dribble well with my left hand. So I was a bit out of joint with my heritage and my peers. You see, athletics is to Alabama as meter is to Shakespeare. Place poor Yorick's skull into the hands of a twelve-year-old Alabama boy and, alas, instead of a eulogy he will deliver a forward pass with it. I was a sophomore in high school before I realized that the Hunchback of Notre Dame was not the university's head coach, Knute Rockne!

My infatuation with the Prince of Denmark probably made me a little weird in high school. One of my English teachers, Mrs. Gates, gave an extra point on our six-week's grade for every twelve lines of poetry we memorized. So Dave Turner and I had a personal contest to see who could learn the most. My old buddy Hamlet came through. I found his two soliloquies, "To be or not to be..." and "So oft it chances in particular men..." made to order. I can remember practicing my delivery, adopting a pensive mood with a Laurence Olivier affectation (his movie "Hamlet" came along about that time), lamenting the torturous inner struggles of young manhood.

Even my mother thought I was taking life a little too seriously. Her family, the Engleberts, were a more genteel version of my father's: humble, Christian-to-the-core, kind, and supportive. In contrast to my father's side, four out of seven of her siblings achieved college degrees and went into teaching professions. All could be described as "reserved" except for Uncle Ben, who was anything but. He was famous for his outrageously obvious toupee of thirty-years' vintage and his penchant for hyperbole. He always arrived late for family reunions on the Fourth of July, making a grand entrance wearing a red-white-and-blue striped blazer and hat. We would all implore him not to doff the hat so we would be spared the toupee, but alas, he would revel in the rebuke. He was the same Uncle Ben who helped pay my mother's way through college when he could barely feed himself. It was a most loving and giving family, and tears come as I write of them. Maybe I have a compassionate Englebert gene in me that carries a DNA pattern linked to the gentle arts of psychiatry (a shrink-link?).

There's something missing in this story, though, regarding my career choice. Medical students choose their specialties for many reasons, often multiple reasons. Sometimes it has to do with temperament (*vide supra*), or identification with mentors, or perks of the trade (such as income, time off, working conditions). I know an orthopedic surgeon who mostly wanted to be the team physician for his college football team. The choice may also have to do with personal or family medical history. I've seen oncologists who were first cancer survivors, and neurologists with epilepsy. Well, what about psychiatrists with their own problems?

Since I am unveiling my life, I may as well tell all. If I'm serious about this thesis that I have been recovering along with Dale, then I can't go halfway. I can't expect Dale to reveal his story without being willing to tell mine. And my story includes a brush with psychiatry as a teen-ager.

I was sixteen years old when I was admitted to the psychiatric ward at Jefferson-Hillman Hospital in Birmingham. Dr. Frank Kay was one of only a handful of psychiatrists in the entire state, so I suspect he was a very busy man. Not too busy to evaluate a troubled teen-ager who had threatened suicide, but too busy to keep him in the hospital very long. My two or three days there are not detailed in my memory, but I do recall some very disturbed-looking people. Probably I was the youngest one there. Dr. Kay, his students, and the staff were kind and gentle. I told my story, and it must not have impressed them much.

It surely impressed my family, though. When I came tearing into the house at midday, crying and hysterical, declaring my disdain for this life, going for the pistol that my sister Mary Lou promptly took from me, they noticed. Not in a mood to respond to entreaties from either Mary Lou or Mother, I ran to the mountain nearby. There I crouched in a canopy of trees and silence, protecting myself from the world I was trying to escape. I didn't know it at the time, but the police had been called to look for me. I planned to sit it out, maybe for days, maybe until I starved to death, believing the pain I could endure there was easier than the pain I had fled. But, alas, my "native hue of resolution [was] sicklied o'er with the pale cast of [rainfall]." A sudden summer shower brought me to a conclusion: I wasn't cut out for martyrdom, at least not of the soggy variety. Sheepishly, I returned home, only a few muddy blocks away, put on dry clothes, and faced the music.

Dad had come home by then and resumed his role in the drama. It was he who had set off the spark for my gesture, with an encounter at his place of business, a drive-in restaurant in the neighborhood where I was working. Some critical remark of his was enough to ignite my waiting tinder-box, and I was off to the races.

The incident was kept very quiet. So quiet, in fact, that my then-four-year-old baby sister, Pat, never knew of it until I began writing this book. It was never spoken of again, until now. When Pat recently began to question my mother about the incident, she somewhat reticently agreed to remove the lid from this family secret and discuss it for the first time. She was able to describe just how distressed about me my father was, and that it was he who had taken the initiative to call Dr. Grote, the family doctor, who had arranged for my psychiatric evaluation.

The upshot was that Dr. Kay pronounced me a rather normal teen-ager who wasn't sure of his father's love, and who had been under a lot of pressure the previous school year. At Dr. Kay's suggestion, Dad committed himself to spending more time with me. This translated into the first of several neat bass-fishing trips to Lake Kissimmee, Florida. Uncle Soup usually went with us, and he managed to show off his wares liberally on these trips; the cooler always went south full of whiskey and north full of fish. His motto seemed to be, "Nature abhors an empty cooler." I really appreciated those trips. They were like initiation rites to manhood. I thank my parents for caring enough to take a very bold step (à la 1952) to get help for me.

So there you have it: Put all this together with the fact that my Professor of Psychiatry at Vanderbilt, Dr. Billy Orr, was a jewel of a person who showed a lot of personal interest in us students, and I've exhausted what I know about my calling to psychiatry. Except that I know I had misgivings about it.

Which brings me back to why I decided to take up mental health center psychiatry. At least a good hunk of the unaccounted-for ninety-percent of my decision must have been a "make-up" job. I was making up — to whom? My father, probably. Making up — for what? For not being what I thought he wanted me to be. For not being as tough or as athletic as he was. For being a psychiatrist. If I could have picked up the baton left on the turf by my politically retired father, I could have run the race for him a little further. I also could have proved that I had made it into the "other world" of downtown, from the other side of the tracks.

It was ironic that the Mental Health Center's first location was in a building directly across the street from First Methodist Church! An incident occurred there that, in retrospect, capsulized much of this dissonance in my life, the conflicting questions within me: Was I a tough kid from the village or an educated professional from the city? Was I my father's or my mother's child? In Eastern terms, it might be described as reconciling my yin and yang. In nineties parlance, I was integrating my Wild Man's soul.

The incident went like this: A schizophrenic patient whom I had treated came into my office unannounced and assaulted me. I protected myself and wrestled him to the floor without striking him back. Since he did not give evidence of being acutely psychotic, and would not explain his actions even to the police when they arrived, I pressed charges. When our court date arrived, the city judge hearing the case happened to be an old high school acquaintance of mine. During the proceedings, he called me to the bench, leaned over, winked at me, and whispered with a twinkle in his eye, "Tell me, Billy, did you hit him back? A Dallas Village boy wouldn't let him get away with that!" He chuckled, and I chuckled. No, I didn't hit him back. This Dallas Village boy had moved into town.

If this sounds like a psychiatrist analyzing himself, it is. This is all hindsight, you know. In 1969 when I joined the Huntsville-Madison County Mental Health Center, I felt aglow with the excitement of a new venture and what I interpreted as altruistic motives vis-à-vis my homefolks. Not until the bottom fell out about ten years later would I be forced to reexamine all this. Some would say I could have avoided a few of these traumas with a good dose of psychoanalysis while I was in training. Such was certainly available to me in Boston. Maybe they are right. Maybe I could have worked through the self-image/father tangle, which could have changed some career decisions and/or behavioral anomalies. And maybe Hamlet could have used it, too. But he didn't, and I didn't.

Today, I also know that there was an even larger reason for my decision to become a psychiatrist. For right now, suffice it to say that my life to this point lacked cohesion and was driven by a dissonance that could not be resolved by my efforts alone. It's a good thing Dale didn't know all this about me at the time. He might have suggested, quite smugly, that I first heal myself and then give him a call. He may have found yet another excuse to postpone recovery.

But that decision was not in his hands.

CHAPTER

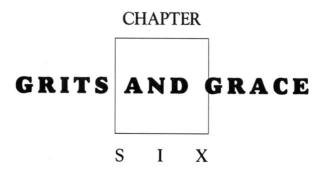

GRITS AND GRACE

S I X

Meanwhile, Dale was still working his way through the stages of alcoholism and manic-depression. Thankfully, we had less of the latter to deal with, and the former was approaching a denouement.

In his last year as a practicing alcoholic (1986), Dale took up a new career. Teaching had lost its zip during a stint with remedial math students at a local high school, so he set his sights on the law enforcement field again. This time he talked his way into the county court house. He even told the judge about his drinking problem, which he allegedly had "under control." The progressive judge decided he would take a chance on Dale, as long as Dale understood he couldn't drink on duty. No problem. You may be getting the picture by now that Dale is a highly competent individual who could probably sell oil to Saddam Hussein.

Dale was hired as a juvenile probation officer on the night shift at the county detention home. But, sales pitch aside, alcohol was clearly still exercising control over his life. A narrative written by Dale, just a few months after the described incident actually occurred, conveys most compellingly the obsessive nature of his preoccupation with drinking. His whole life revolved around the next drink: when he could have it and how he could assure its availability:

Friday, October 10, 1986, 10:30 p.m.

Mary Lou shakes me awake and tells me it is time to go to work. We start a conversation about making the coffee, but I'm not listening — too busy with my usual mental inventory — vodka, ice, cups, mix. When I get off work at 8 a.m., it is impossible to find a liquor store or bar open, and besides, I need a drink as soon as I hit the courthouse parking lot at the end of my shift. Just yesterday I forgot to get some ice from the drug testing laboratory at the detention home to put in the Ziplock baggies stashed in my briefcase. The twenty-four hour market provided a source of ice, but who needs ten pounds for an eight-ounce tumbler? And several times I have forgotten the plastic cup and ended up buying a package of fifty paper cups and depositing forty-nine in the trash can outside the store.

I jump in the shower and wake up enough to run through the check list, stopping at VODKA. Where will I find a bottle? Before going to bed, I finished the one in my briefcase. I know there must be five or six quarts hidden in the house, but finding them with Mary Lou around is a real trick. If she weren't sitting in the recreation room, I could sneak to the bar and lift a bottle from there. I wonder to myself if she watches TV by the bar instead of upstairs just to keep me from the liquor supply. Does she know I'm taking liquor to my job?

I pray she doesn't follow me to the garage. Then I can unlock the hunting cabinet and look for hidden treasure. She doesn't, so I breathe a sigh of relief as I feel the familiar glass shape in one of my hip boots in the cabinet. What a clever guy I am, with all my stashes! Into my briefcase goes the bottle, and I check once more for all the essentials — baggie for ice, tumbler, sixteen-ounce bottle of 7-Up with screw top.

I haven't had a drink for seven hours, and the shakes will be here in less than four more. Tonight is Friday, and the police will probably bring in several juveniles, hopefully only the usual drunk brats. I can handle that with only three forms to complete. But it's those damn felonies with nine different forms to fill out and sign! If they bring in two carloads, I'll be shaking too hard to sign all the papers before I'm done. Just last Saturday I didn't finish papers until 3 a.m., and my signature was barely legible!

Starting my shift, I check the mail and finish whatever paperwork is there, before the shakes start. Uh-oh! There's a bit of bad news in the mail. My supervisor left a memo asking me to run the tests on four urine specimens in the refrigerator. Last week I waited too long to do that, and I was shaking so bad the pipette sounded like the triangle in a rhythm band, hitting the side of the test tube. Tonight I'll get it done earlier.

Glancing at my watch, I see that it's now 5:15 a.m., less than three hours now til I can drink again! Then – oh crap! – here comes another black and white, and I recognize the kid in handcuffs as a repeater felon. And here come those nine forms. The way my coffee is shaking, I know my signature will be hopeless. I hold the key with two hands to open the door and let them in. After checking the kid in, searching him, and bedding him down, I set myself to the task. Typing the reports as rapidly as my palsy will allow, I then practice my signature on scrap paper. No good! Totally illegible! I search for other options. Maybe I can wait until the next night and finish them. No, the judge will want to handle this case before Sunday, so I have to finish them.

The next option is the obvious solution. The way to stop shaking is to take a drink. If I'm caught, it will be curtains for the job. The judge's words ring in my ears: "If we ever smell alcohol on you, you will be terminated immediately." But at this point I don't have a choice, so I open my briefcase and remove the necessary items. I fill the cup with ice and add the vodka and 7-Up. A quick look out the windows to see if the coast is clear, and down the hatch. After a few minutes I check my signature again – still a little shaky – so I pour another tumbler full and drink it. Soon I'm fit to sign the Declaration of Independence.

The next shift will be arriving soon, so I carefully place my paraphernalia back in the briefcase and pop a few Certs in my mouth. When they arrive, I keep a cautious distance, make up some story about being in a hurry to go fishing, and leave. This morning I don't have to follow my drink-in-the-parking-lot routine, since I've already had one. Instead, I drive a few blocks, pull over to the side, and set up the bar. As I sit by the side of the road, I go over my mental shopping list for the day. First, it's the liquor store, then a supermarket for baggies, 7-Up, and Certs. I will probably just have to drink on duty again. Probably even tonight!

Two weeks before this episode, I had seen Dale for an appointment, and he had told me then that he was drinking heavily. I had suggested he go into the hospital for detox and treatment, but he had put it off. Finally, ten days after this episode, he agreed to go in.

It had been over six years since I had gotten that first call from Suzanne at Crestwood Hospital. Six years of uncertain expectancy. But this was to be a different experience than his prior hospital encounters, and thank God for that.

Dale does thank God, indeed. Though he didn't tell us at the time, he had experienced a life-changing event just before coming into the hospital. He had spent the weekend holed up by himself in a Holiday Inn, drinking. That, in itself, was not unusual. One time he drove all the way to a Holiday Inn near the Rio Grande and totaled his car in Mexico on one of his solo adventures. This time, though, he stayed around town; he just didn't tell Mary Lou where he was. When he woke on Sunday, his mind a blur about the events of the previous twenty-four hours, he opened the motel door to see where he was and to wake himself up. His Buick was parked where he could see it, and what he saw shocked him. There was a dent in the left front fender. He had no recollection, of course, of anything happening, having been in an alcoholic blackout all evening. But there was enough of a dent that it was obviously made by a significant encounter with some object. Yet there was no paint gone and no foreign paint from another car. In fact, it looked like the sort of dent that would be caused by striking a large animal — or person!

> *The thoughts of this grew in my mind and became more and more oppressive. I paced in my room, looking again at the car through the window to confirm what I had seen. Had I struck someone? Could I have severely injured — or killed — someone and not recall a damn thing about it? Suddenly, I was overwhelmed by fear and guilt. What was happening to my life? Was this the way I was supposed to be? Was there any help for me?*

> *And with that, I collapsed to my knees in that motel room, weeping and praying to a God I had tried to forget for a long time. I prayed out loud, asking for God's presence in my life and some direction to guide me out of the living death I was going through.*

As Dale recounted that episode, I felt a great empathy with him. I had come to my own desperate moment a few years earlier, 1978 to be exact, when my professional life had come apart with my departure from the Huntsville-Madison County Mental Health Center. Flushed with pain and confusion, I had left my last meeting of the board of directors and arrived home in an emotional blackout. My realizations were not as time-condensed and dramatic as were Dale's; i.e., I didn't get on my knees at that time, at least not literally. But figuratively I did, as I began the slow climb out of that spiritless slough.

Dale believes very firmly that God answered his prayer. Soon after that motel morning he was in Crestwood Hospital again, more humble and submissive than ever before. He accepted my refusal to give him Antabuse anymore, or to send him home after detox, or to bypass the AA Program. He even accepted my suggestion (shall we say insistence?) that he receive extended treatment at a recovery center in Minnesota.

Dale had heard the words "Hazelden," "Minnesota," and "extended rehabilitation" before. He had some misgivings about the "extended" part and really didn't know much about Hazelden. I explained that this place was considered a pioneer in the treatment of chemical dependency and was internationally respected in the field of rehabilitation. Some categorize it with another Minnesota colossus, calling it the "Mayo Clinic of Alcoholism." Dale agreed to go.

I wasted no time getting things under way.

"Vern, this is Bill Goodson down in Huntsville, Alabama. How's it going up there in Lake Wobegon, brother?"

I was calling Vern Wagner at the Hazelden Foundation in Center City, Minnesota. He didn't have anything to do with new admissions, but I knew him personally, and when you're calling a foreign country like that, it helps to hear a familiar voice on the other end. I had gotten to know Vern when he had come down to Alabama on a two-day mission to consult with us — a group of four mental health professionals

— on how to set up an outpatient chemical dependency program. It was instant chemistry with Vern and us, topped off by a breakfast meeting at Eunice's Country Kitchen where he learned to lust (love is too tame) for country ham, grits, red-eye gravy, and biscuits.

When visitors come to Huntsville, I love to take them to Eunice's place. It is so down-home that even the chairs squeak "y'all." Breakfast at Eunice's is a local custom for all sorts of folks, mainly because Eunice Merrell keeps you coming back with her smiles and hugs, but also because she serves up a mean plate of Southern fare. Many Yankees, like Vern, are puzzled when they see the blob of white grainy substance next to their eggs. They will often ask, "What's that? I don't think I ordered it." To which the reply comes, "In the South, grits just come, you don't have to order them." Some say grits and God's grace have a lot in common.

Another reason I like to patronize Eunice's is that it is located in the mill village where I was born, and I feel at home there. Many of the old-timers are friends of my parents, and a host of memories await me with each visit. But I stray...

"I've got a patient," I explained to Vern, "who's agreed to come there for treatment, a native Minnesotan, no less! But he's been in Alabama so long that he doesn't wear shoes anymore, has forgotten how to talk, and thinks Republicans are people who associate with some kind of sinners that Jesus talked about. So if we're going to send him up there, we need a head start to give him a crash course in civilization and speaking Minnesotan."

After a minute or two of such good-natured bantering and Vern's inquiry as to Eunice's health, we got down to business. He connected me with the admissions officer, who cordially and efficiently set up the admission procedure for Dale. Luckily, their waiting list was only a week or two.

I was savoring the moment, hardly believing that Dale was actually agreeing to this. He seemed so different this time, not dismissing the AA Program out of hand. I had talked to him about Hazelden many times before, but he had always had a wisecrack and a ready smile to cast the notion aside. What was happening? You see, Dale had not divulged to me his experience at the motel — probably because he didn't think I would believe him. In fact, it was only when we sat down to begin writing this book together that he shared with me his story of the morning that had provoked such a change in him.

Not wont to look gift horses in the mouth, I didn't press Dale for the reasons for his new-found humility. I simply accepted it as a blessing and kept him at Crestwood until his number came up at Hazelden. Many of us were excited about this. For years, Bob R. and I had tried to send patients to Hazelden; that had always been our backup plan for patients who failed repeatedly at local treatment. Some might say that we threatened patients with Hazelden; I say we offered it. But in all those years, we never had a "done deal." Sometimes the finances weren't there, but most often the patient just wasn't willing to go so far away. An alcoholic will use any excuse to avoid recovery, so eleven hundred miles and visions of fifteen-foot snowdrifts turned into convincing obstacles for most of our reluctant patients.

But all this seemed interesting to Dale — something good about Minnesota for a change! (The Twins and Vikings weren't much good at that time.) Center City — Dale hadn't heard of that small town in almost forty years. It is only twenty-five miles or so from where he grew up. The last time he had been there had been with a group of young people from his church. They had had a picnic and a softball tournament and had visited the oldest Lutheran church in Minnesota. What an ironic fate, Dale thought. He had traveled, by vocation or vacation, to Japan, Canada, Mexico, most of the Caribbean, and almost all of the United States, living in the West and in the South. And now we were recommending that he go home to recover! Sort of like someone telling me I had to go back to Epworth Methodist Church to find my salvation!

From that point on Dale recalls that he was neither reluctant nor zealous about the transfer. He was surrendering to his destiny. Although he did not understand it at the time, Dale believes that God was directing his life. From the moment he had gotten up off his knees in that motel room, he believed he had lost the compulsion to drink alcohol. And even though he was convinced, truly for the first time, that he would never drink again, he acquiesced to the trip north.

On the drive from the airport in Minneapolis to Hazelden, reality seemed to dawn. Dale realized he was going to be a thousand miles from home and family for several months. Surprisingly, he was not perturbed, even in light of his numerous hospitalizations and treatments in the past. This time he was ready, willing, and able. He firmly believed this was to be the last time in treatment for him.

Traveling the short distance through Center City, Dale saw the old Lutheran church, a majestic remembrance, pass by on his left. Another mile or two down the road, he was recollecting the approach to his very first treatment in Atlanta more than six years prior. Then, the large brick buildings had loomed ominous, while the lifeless grounds had seemed to precipitate gloom. What he saw on this occasion was quite different. The mile-long ride across Hazelden's two-hundred-fifty acres of hills, woods, and fields surrounded by colorful autumn flora and fauna made an initial impression that helps to explain why Hazelden attracts and keeps people. Even more important than the physical layout, though, was the aura of serenity that permeated the place.

Dale began incorporating some of that serenity right away, as he was learning to "accept those things I cannot change" — such as Hazelden's requirement that he spend twenty-four hours in the detox unit, and that Mary Lou not accompany him after she checked him in. The old Dale would have argued and cajoled: After all, he had just spent two weeks in detox at Crestwood, and his wife had come all that distance and now was being asked to turn around and fly away! The new Dale surrendered. He stayed, and Mary Lou went back to Alabama.

After the staff was assured he was not going into alcohol withdrawal, Dale began attending AA meetings, a ritual that was to continue during his stay. How ironic it was that the first meeting he visited was in the basement of — you guessed it — the old Center City Lutheran Church of his youth! Even more meaningful was the discussion topic for that meeting: "Dry and Sober." That meeting is still very vivid for Dale. He remembers a couple of AA old-timers philosophizing that if recovery were just not-drinking, it would be very easy. One of them joked, "Just find a policeman and give him a bloody nose. You'll get thirty days without drinking, but that ain't sobriety." Dale had no trouble relating to this example, thinking of his belief that he was recovered because he entered Crestwood without a compulsion to use alcohol. Another milestone discovery: Not drinking is just the beginning of sobriety; sobriety is just the beginning of recovery.

Dale was amazed as the days went by. People were recovering

emotionally, physically, mentally, and spiritually. His own progress, he could not judge as clearly, but he sensed he was undergoing progressive character change. To explain what happened to him, he says, would be as difficult as explaining such nebulous concepts as heaven or love. He can only share what he perceived and the effect it had on his life.

Hazelden was, for Dale, a big twenty-four-hour-a-day AA meeting with short breaks and sleep. It was an amalgam of devotion, emotion, and inspiration, where every assembly started with a moment of silence and the Serenity Prayer and closed with holding hands, the Lord's Prayer, and hugs. (Yes – hugs! Another milestone: Not only is it okay for men to cry, it is acceptable for them to hug each other.) The spirituality of the Twelve Steps, along with the reawakening of associations with his Lutheran background, pulled Dale toward a renewal of his spirit. He began to examine the nature of his relationship to himself, others, and his Higher Power.

This was being accomplished in a community of peers. During his months at Hazelden, Dale roomed with Peter T., an attorney about the same age as Dale's deceased brother, Curtis. The two got along exceedingly well, becoming close friends; and Dale cultivated a confidant to replace Curtis, as he and Peter shared lengthy, serious dialogue on a daily basis, often late into the night. They shared their prior and developing spirituality, as well as their hopes and dreams. Within this friendship Dale was experiencing the kind of relationship, similar to working with a sponsor, that is so strongly recommended by AA, where the AA member chooses a more experienced one to be a mentor. Dale couldn't help but wish, as he often still does, that Curtis could have experienced the recovery in AA that he was as he reached out to his peers among his new-found brothers and sisters.

At Hazelden, Dale developed a genuine appreciation for the simple but profound principles of the AA Program. He knew that, with a dedicated effort to attend meetings and study the literature, he could acquire the rudiments of the Program and understand how it works.

In the meantime, I was getting regular monthly reports from the staff, regarding Dale's progress. Most of them were glowing in their praise of his efforts. Occasionally, I would see remarks as to his ego and defensiveness. But, overall, I was breathing much easier, given what I was hearing.

Then the bombshell came. I got a call from his counselor with the distressing news that Dale was refusing to stay any longer, despite the staff's recommendations. "Oh, no! Dale's back to his old tricks," I thought.

I didn't try to talk to him and persuade him otherwise. In fact, he was already on his way home. Since he was still on lithium and needed an aftercare monitor, the Hazelden staff had instructed him to call me for a follow-up appointment. I anxiously awaited my first interview with him, praying he hadn't fallen off the wagon already.

My fears melted away after that first meeting. He was truly a different Dale, totally immersed in the AA Program, attending meetings every day, and spouting the lingo. He had more cliches than Bob R.! He explained to me his reasons for leaving Hazelden against advice. Quite simply, it boiled down to the fact that he now had confidence in his dedication to recovery. The compulsion to drink had never returned since the motel incident, and he had an extraordinary faith that God was with him. Incidentally, he admitted, he also didn't want to spend more time and money on the project. (Dale has always had a well-honed pecuniary sense.)

Lest this chapter begin to sound like a marketing ploy for the Hazelden Foundation, let me put things in perspective. There are many first-class treatment centers in our country, and miraculous things happen in them every day. Not all of them are as totally AA in their philosophy as is Hazelden, and staffing patterns vary. It is clear, however, that with Dale, Hazelden was the right choice. As he puts it, "Just like the Chicago Cubs' legendary double-play trio, Tinkers-to-Evers-to Chance, my winning play was Crestwood-to-Hazelden-to-AA."

Dale was beginning to understand what the Big Book of Alcoholics Anonymous meant, that he could "know a new freedom and a new happiness, as well as a realization that God was doing for him what he could not do for himself." He was now entering the third phase of his life; he had moved from nondrinking, to drinking, into healthy recovery.

CHAPTER

GOD'S TIME

S E V E N

Life is only for Love.
Time is only that we may find God.
–St. Bernard

How many times have you wondered to yourself, "Would it have made a difference if...?" As in, "If I had bought that stock a month later when it was down five, would it still be up ten now?" Or, as in the time I arrived at the Vanderbilt versus Auburn football game a minute after kickoff and Vanderbilt was already seven points behind. What if I had been there on time? Would my cheering or banner-waving have somehow caused the safety to line up a little closer to the line of scrimmage so that he would have made the touchdown-stopping tackle? Or how about the first time I saw a beautiful, long-blond-haired girl visiting her grandmother in Huntsville one summer in 1950, and I knew I *had* to be introduced to her. What if I hadn't gone to the swimming pool that day? Would I have seen my wife-to-be somewhere else, or would our future lives be totally different without that chance encounter? And what about the fact that it was my own sister who introduced us a few days hence, without my provocation? A happy coincidence?

We all experience similar "what if's" in our lives, from apparently inconsequential circumstances, such as stock prices, to life-directing events, such as meeting our mate. Sometimes these are dramatic, time-compressed occurrences that, in their very nature, resound throughout the rest of our lives. Sometimes sudden tragic events defy us to discount them and leave us with a sense of destiny and wonder. I think of the tornado that hit Huntsville in 1989. Some twenty people lost their lives within that few minutes of nature's wrath. There were tales by the hundreds of individuals who were near-misses, like that of a housewife who had delayed her shopping trip a few minutes and thereby avoided the devastated shopping center.

Our lives are full of coincidences: chance happenings that can lead to dramatic events or nonevents. My point is to stir up your thinking about events or chains of events in your life — and their consequences. Why do I want to do this? Because it will help put into perspective the encounter between Dale and me, and our encounter with God.

I believe Dale would have recovered without me. I believe Auburn would have scored that touchdown on the first play from scrimmage whether I had been there or not, and in that particular case I infer no lasting consequences for my life. With Dale, however, I would have missed a great deal by not participating in his recovery, even if I wasn't a required ingredient for his success.

I seem to be saying very opposite things; namely, that we do make a difference . . . and we don't. That the chance happenings as well as the deliberate choices and decisions are important determinants in our lives, and yet all will come out the same regardless of these things. It would seem we can't have it both ways. But I think we can — depending on our perspective about the things that matter in this world.

For instance, one thing that matters is *outcome*. The end results of events are important — results like sobriety, a happy marriage, a win on the football field. There is no denying that *the way things turn out* means a lot to us. Yet, *the way we get there* matters, too. The decisions we make, the mistakes from which we learn, the lives we touch and influence — these processes form the miracles of life that provide color and richness to existence. The whips and scorns of time, as well as the joys that pass understanding, are the stuff that the full life is made of. They form the crucible in which the ore of our youth is refined to the purer metal of maturity. By alchemy or chemistry, by hook or by crook, by the grace of God, we come to where we are.

In all of this, the people we meet and the influence we have on each other make a difference. Encounters with other human beings create the true and lasting learning experiences. And I believe that God works through us and for us when we are in a position to make choices that facilitate the turning points in our lives.

For Dale, the turning point was the motel experience. Without that experience, he might not have humbled himself to ask God's help and submitted to the treatment he needed. I've asked myself many times whether the moment could have been hastened by different choices on my part, or Mary Lou's part, or somebody's. But puzzling over that isn't very meaningful in the long run because things happen in God's time, not ours.

God's time? What's that?

I'll digress for a moment. My wife and I are Episcopalians. The Episcopal Church has adopted a program from the Roman Catholics called Cursillo (which is Spanish for "short course"). Cursillo is a renewal-type movement involving an intensive, highly structured, three-day weekend experience followed by weekly follow-up meetings in small groups, called Reunion Groups. When my wife and I arrived for our Cursillo retreat, we were asked to surrender our watches or other timepieces to the staff, with the announcement that we would be on "God's time" for the weekend. At first that seemed rather dramatic and overdone to me. But its meaning became very significant as we learned to give ourselves to the process of the weekend, in essence to give up control of our time and submit to whatever happened.

To say that this weekend was a most compelling experience to me would be an understatement, but to elaborate more would distract from the present agenda. Suffice it to say that by accepting God's time, I was acknowledging my own powerlessness over my life without God's direction. By acknowledging this, I was preparing myself to be ready for what God was to bring to me *whenever* it was to happen. God's time means "not my will, but thine be done." It also means that I cannot see the big picture. I don't know when things are going to come together, to coalesce at the precise time that they do. I had best give up my timepiece, take my time, and time will tell. And, in the meantime, be guided by my best instincts and pay attention to what's happening.

Paying attention, learning, and growing are the main points. In the practice of psychiatry (or medicine), it is tempting to adopt a different posture in relationship to patients; namely to "be in charge" and to assume that, because we are physicians, we should always know better and more than our patients. Dr. Bernie Segal has spoken eloquently to this point in his book *Love, Medicine, and Miracles* from the point of view of the surgeon, who is supposed to epitomize the god-complex often attributed to the medical profession. He sets an example of openness and dialogue that enriches the doctor-patient relationship.

I know I have learned from my relationships with alcoholic patients. I know I have learned from my encounter with Dale.

By this point in my work with Dale, I had grown in my clinical abilities, in the diagnosing of dual-diagnosis patients. I had learned something about the orchestration of treatment for such complex patients. More subtly, I was learning about God's time: to be patient, do my best, and follow my hunches, long enough for something to happen that turns the tide. The business of hunches (or intuitions, more properly) is quite to the point here. Straight textbook management may have told me to draw the line on Dale much sooner in his treatment — to desist from prescribing Antabuse, to refuse to see him unless he submitted to meaningful treatment. And I have done that in other cases. In Dale's case, though, I followed my intuitions and played out the line instead of trying to muscle him in. Any angler knows you don't muscle in a ten-pound bass on a four-pound test line. And even though you never know the exact weight of the fish until it's in the boat, there are hunches about it, which guide the reeling intensity. So it was with Dale and me — the difference being that he was one of the most savvy fishes in the pond and almost outwitted himself.

God was playing the line with me at the same time. When my tenure as a mental health center psychiatrist had come to an abrupt and unpleasant end in 1979, I had placed myself in a searching mode regarding my spiritual life. I had bottomed out and was feeling rather desperate. I felt betrayed, unappreciated, angry, ashamed, alone, you name it. Mostly, though, I grieved the loss of a large part of my professional life and ambition that had consumed my energies for a decade. I had felt satisfaction in returning to my hometown and helping to start a comprehensive mental health center. It had seemed "made to order" — except for one thing: I was allowing it to lead me further and further into the myth of self-reliance.

I don't mean that I was practicing psychiatry as a loner. On the contrary, I was fulfilling the role of a good team player, working with psychologists, nurses, social workers, counselors; trying to create an environment where all staff had meaningful roles and input into the clinical work. So I wasn't "playing God" vis-à-vis paramedical personnel, in the usual perverted sense of medical parlance. What I was doing was overestimating my importance to the enterprise, to the point that I was blind to the larger realities of the community's agenda.

Unfortunately, I had alienated some highly-placed state mental health officials with my outspoken stance about the funding of community centers. These were GEORGE WALLACE DAYS, folks, when the "good ol' boy" connections decided ninety-nine percent of the funding priorities. Montgomery wasn't too keen about some brash young psychiatrist from Huntsville pointing out the inadequacies of state planning. I cringe as I recall one of my written statements to the effect that Alabama mental health was leaping boldly into the nineteenth century with its plans to build more regional hospitals. I surely believed that my heart was in the right place, that I was looking out for the mentally ill in my community. (Notice all the first-person pronouns?)

I had directed the Mental Health Center into a position of some prominence, offering research and clinical programs that were considered by many to be innovative and effective. We had a talented and enthusiastic staff. But at the point that I became an irritant to state officials, my usefulness to the enterprise began to decline. Several things happened over the period of a couple of years, from 1976 to 1978: I stepped aside as Executive Director to do full-time clinical work; strife among the staff led to polarization around the new Executive Director; and I sided with the anti-Director forces.

Such divisiveness was clearly destructive to the Center's mission. And when my position in it finally gave the powers-that-be the opportunity to buy up my contract, they did so. I imagine it wasn't an easy thing for the Board of Directors to do. After all, I had contributed a lot of time and energy to the development of programs; I was a hometown boy whose father had been prominent in the councils of city government; I wasn't really a bad person. No, mine was the sin of zeal, an addiction to a particular image of my place in the scheme of things. I had become too much identified with the work and had lost a greater vision of proper perspective. I didn't see the Big Picture, which you only get if you remove the blinder of Self and *let things happen*. I hadn't turned my watch in.

Dale and I were reaching bottom at about the same time, he drunk and sick with alcohol; I, with self-importance and pride. Little did I know that this professional crisis in my life would eventually lead me to recovery and renewal, just as Dale's motel experience led him to turn the corner. I came home from my last Mental Health Center Board meeting at which I announced my resignation and dissolved in tears before Willa, my fifteen-year-old daughter, clumsily trying to explain to her why her father was reduced to such a state. She may not have understood to this day, perhaps not until she reads this account.

As Dale put himself in the hands of others, I did, too. I did it in three phases.

First, I pursued in an intentional manner an exploration of things spiritual. Among my friends were many who had considerable religious life, private and public. Some were ministers, others laypersons of theological bent. I picked three of these friends and had private discussions with them. I told them that I felt something was missing in my life, that I had ignored the spiritual part of myself for many years, and that I needed their help. I asked them to offer suggestions as to how I could pursue this quest, and they did.

Clearly, I picked individuals who I thought would be sensitive to my fragile state of need. I did not choose, first, my family, among whom were several deeply devout members. I did not choose them because, just like a patient selecting a therapist, I wanted objectivity in my mentors. Likewise, I did not choose individuals with fundamentalist beliefs; I wasn't likely to be on the same frequency at all, and reverberations of Easter morning and the dear Trance Lady still rang in my head.

Bob Gonia was one of the people I turned to. He was an ordained Methodist minister who had made a second career in administration of social services in our community. I knew, too, that he recently had become the spiritual leader of a small ecumenical "church" group. This was no ordinary church, inasmuch as they met rather informally as a group of twenty or thirty. Bob invited me to attend, which I did on one occasion. It was a congenial group with a shared need for unconventional religious communion. I may have benefited from such a group, but its prospects for continuity seemed tenuous to me, especially when Bob took a position in another city.

Townsend Walker was another of my chosen advisors. I had admired his committed approach to theology as I had observed him at work in the community for several years. He organized and chaired an ongoing series of seminars in Huntsville, called the Vanderbilt Study Forum, wherein faculty of the Vanderbilt University Divinity School would chug down I-65 to conduct evening lectures and discussion groups for interested persons. These programs were very well attended over the years, and I had dropped in on them occasionally. It seemed quaintly ironic that the university which opened my eyes to humanism now offered a path of reentry to theism for me. I also knew that Townsend himself had returned in his middle age to Vanderbilt to obtain an advanced degree in theology. As you might expect, his suggestions for me were oriented primarily toward reading material. His was weighty stuff, the likes of Schweitzer, Bonhoffer, Niebuhr, and Tillich. I plowed through these with dogged determinism, convinced that somehow my mind would begin to assimilate the Ground of My Being with the Historical Jesus.

Emile Joffrion, an Episcopal priest, also honored my request for guidance. He was rector of the venerable Church of the Nativity in downtown Huntsville and a much respected pillar of the community (the local equivalent of Walter Cronkite). My first session with him turned into a combination therapeutic/cathartic and spiritual direction event. He must have been through it a few thousand times in his career, but it was my first. I experienced the power of directed empathic support such as I had never known, having always previously been on the other side of that desk. I poured out my heart to him, ventilating the anger and hurt that was there. He didn't try to vindicate my actions; he simply validated me as a person. The one direct suggestion that came out of that visit was an invitation to visit his church to see if it had anything to offer me.

The real surprise to me was that I didn't reject Emile's invitation out of hand. At this juncture in my quest, I had not at all come to the conclusion that organized religion could be in the picture for me. I guess I was hoping I could absorb something by study, or meditation, or anything short of walking inside a church building, for God's sake!! I knew I was a needy person, but *that* needy?? I had to think that one over awhile.

This began the second phase of my quest; namely, reentry into organized religion. Not only did I have to think it over carefully, but talk it over, too, with my wife, Elise. Through medical school, three daughters, making a home and professional life together (she is a middle-school teacher); through the joys and sorrows of my recent career happenings, she had stood beside me like a rock. She was now to participate with me in this quest, inasmuch as she had always maintained church affiliation with the Methodists and welcomed any sign of my rapprochement. Our daughters, likewise, had been sporadic attenders at my old church home, First Methodist, at least until high school, when they tended to do their own thing. The oldest, Dorothy, actually became the first Episcopalian in the family when, as a teen-ager, she joined the Church of the Nativity to be with some of her closer friends. I had neither dis-nor-encouraged such affiliations; rather, I had been a passive bystander in their religious education. And Elise had tolerated with equanimity all my years of doubt and agnosticism.

She was happy to share in the new venture, as we decided to visit adult Sunday School classes in the two denominations we seemed most drawn to: Methodist and Episcopal. Emile steered me to a particular class in his Episcopal church that was, shall we say, avant-garde. The subject of the class on the 'test' Sunday we visited was a study of Mother Earth symbolism in literature, with comparative and contrasting Christian beliefs. It was a sort of quasireligious anthropology/literature class, led by an outlandishly outspoken teacher, Evie Spearman, who captured my attention with her breadth of knowledge and sharp sense of humor. The discussions from the participants were free-wheeling, conflictual, animated. I thought to myself, "This kind of Christianity, I do not have to flee. Even my views would be tolerated here."

It didn't take Elise and me long to make our decision. My quest entered a new phase as I began a dialogue with others in this new Anglican setting, many whom I already knew, and many who were to become friends and fellow-questors. After a year or so of Sunday-School-only attendance, we then found our way into the church services proper, via the choir loft. It had been many years since we had sung in choir together, but this was a natural entrée to solidify our ties to the church. I am reminded of one of those profound sayings of my old buddy, Bob R. When a new patient would find his way into the hospital sheepishly and unwillingly, Bob would refer to him as having "slithered in by the boiler room." I guess I slithered into the church by the choir loft, feeling just as uncomfortable and uncertain as had Dale on his first trip to Crestwood.

In my surrender to God's Time, I had put myself into the hands of others, just as Dale had. I had searched for and found a community of fellow-questors. But there was a third phase overlapping with the others that was not as focused, more subtle, and yet just as powerful: I opened the door for God's intervention into my working day. I began listening to and observing my patients differently; I began to allow their spiritual lives and mine to creep into the therapy sessions.

Most of us have to make a living in the secular world. We can't all be saints, or monks, or clergypersons. The followers of St. Francis of Assisi realized that when they established the Third Order. The First Franciscan Order was the Friars Minor, who lived under the Rule of St. Francis, gave up worldly possessions, became monks, and traveled the byroads of the Umbrian countryside in Italy. The Second Order was the distaff side, the Poor Clairs. The Third Order, however, was comprised of everyday men and women who maintained worldly connections but practiced the virtues of the Rule within the limits of their circumstances. As G.K. Chesterton put it, "The Third Order... was designed to assist ordinary men to be ordinary with an extraordinary exultation." No less figures than St. Louis, Dante, and Galvani were counted among the members of this dedicated group of mostly ordinary mortals who yearned for the devoted life that marked St. Francis and his roving band. It was their aspiration to impregnate the patchwork of their daily lives with the stuff that saints are made of; to weave threads of holiness into the fabric of profession and commerce.

Could I aspire to be a Third-Order type? In my profession there is a range of opinion as to the propriety of incorporating religious aspects into one's practice. At the one pole are the stereotypical atheists who treat religious sentiments in their patients as quasi-pathological manifestations. At the other pole are some so-called "Christian psychiatrists" who participate in healing services, pray regularly with their patients, and use scriptural references in a therapeutic context. I believe most psychiatrists are in the middle ground, acknowledging the importance of religion for many of their patients, but not apt to credit mystical experiences with a great deal of therapeutic benefit. As I worked with Dale and his peers in this metamorphic decade of my life, I found myself shifting to the right of center.

I became more and more comfortable acknowledging that my patients found strength in faith and prayer. This came somewhat easily since I was seeing many alcoholic patients who were being led to spiritual renewal in their Twelve-Step recovery programs! There was no need to force conversation in that direction; every day in the hospital was beginning with a meditation; the Lord's Prayer was repeated regularly at meetings; and the Serenity Prayer was posted on walls everywhere.

In fact, if I didn't engage the patient in conversation about the Higher Power concept, I was not in step with the process of therapy at all. I was blessed with an inundation of opportunity to practice what I hadn't preached in a long time: that the patient and I were engaged in a journey together, to find strength beyond ourselves to heal what was broken.

It wasn't long before my new-found comfort with alcoholics began to work its way into my relationships with other types of patients. I couldn't be quite as bold in spiritual talk with the general adult psychiatry patients I saw in my practice because they weren't being "tuned up" that way in self-help groups. But many of them expressed spiritual concerns, and I was able to respond comfortably. I often found that there was a spiritual void in their lives, and I was able to ease into that topic without fear of treading on foreign soil because the soil wasn't foreign to me anymore. I was able to share some of my own experiences, at the appropriate times.

Just for fun, imagine a hypothetical generic clinical interview situation and compare what my responses would have been at various points in my career. The patient, let's say, is a forty-five-year-old recently divorced engineer who is depressed, lonely, and angry with almost everyone. This is my second session with him, and he is still a somewhat reluctant participant in therapy, mainly because he believes he should be able to handle his problems himself.

Patient: *"Sometimes I'm not sure what life is all about, anyway."*

Me: *"How do you mean?"*

Patient: *"Well, you know, whether there's any purpose to it — to my life."*

Me: "That must be a pretty bad feeling; tell me more about it."

Patient: "Oh, I don't know . . . I wonder if there's a God, and, if so, what difference that makes for me."

(Dialogue continues now in three different time frames.)

TIME FRAME I:
1963, PSYCHIATRIC RESIDENCY

Me: "Sometimes it's easier to place the problem 'way out there' or to blame someone not within reach, rather than deal with the here and now."

Patient: [testily] "I don't think that's what I'm doing."

Me: [evenly] "Maybe we can take a look at that . . ."

(Note: Patient doesn't return for third appointment and never pays the bill.)

TIME FRAME II:
1975, MENTAL HEALTH CENTER DAYS

Me: "You're asking some good questions, questions that bother a lot of patients. Spiritual matters are important, but maybe not the best way for us to use our time together. Perhaps your pastor could be of help to you there. I'll be glad to talk with your minister if you like."

Patient: [a bit puzzled] "Oh, okay, I see what you mean."

(Note: Patient doesn't return but does pay the bill.)

TIME FRAME III:
THE PRESENT

Me: *"You know, I'm glad you put it that way. I sort of suspected you were struggling some with your spiritual life; and even though I'm not a spiritual director, I can see your need to explore this some more. We all go through times of doubt and fear."*

Patient: *"You mean it's all right to talk about God in here? I thought psychiatrists were generally anti-that sort of thing."*

Me: *"That's a common stereotype — just like the one that says engineers are nonfeeling people, but you and I know that one isn't so, right? Well, neither is the one about psychiatrists. Now, I don't plan to have a revival meeting in here with you, but I'm sure open to talking with you about a part of you that is extremely important. So don't worry; if I get in over my head, I'll let you know."*

(Note: He came back, and he paid.)

It would not be uncommon, as I got to know this patient, for me to share with him some of my own history, to inquire more about his organized religious attachment, and to make suggestions for strengthening them. All of this can be interspersed smoothly with the other issues in therapy, without compromising the therapeutic relationship. As I have done this, I have been able to feel more integrated, myself, and have enjoyed a more authentic experience with patients. I'm not treading barefoot in my brown sackcloth on the backroads of Umbria, searching for lepers to hug, but I do feel a little closer to a Third Order calling.

Speaking of monks, I am reminded of another patient who helped to ignite a genuine flame in me. Also an alcoholic, Brian (not his real name) was in treatment at Crestwood, and we were having some lively discussions about religion. An erstwhile Roman Catholic who had, in his earlier years, aspired to the priesthood, he had fallen away and was groping back. Needless to say, I tuned in easily. I had been reading Henri Nouwen's *Genessee Diary*, with which Brian was quite familiar. In this book Nouwen relates his experience of being on a lengthy retreat at a Trappist monastery in New York State. It is a captivating narrative, as he relates the joys and hardships of the contemplative life. Nouwen's candor regarding his own shortcomings is refreshing and touched a special chord with me at the time. As a corollary to our discussions, Brian introduced me to the writings of Thomas Merton, informing me that Merton had become a Trappist monk at the Abbey of Gethsemani, a monastery near Bardstown, Kentucky.

When I looked at the map and saw that Bardstown was a mere five-hour drive from my hometown, the urge came upon me to make a visit there. A call to the guestmaster, Brother Luke, led to the first of several weekend retreats I was to make to the abbey. A group of interested men usually leave Huntsville around twelve noon on Friday, and we return on Sunday afternoon. The quiet depth of God's presence in that place is almost indescribable. That fortuitous encounter with Brian has made a profound influence on my life, and I often tell him of my gratitude.

When I begin to open myself up to spiritual dialogue, and especially if I share my personal experiences, a door is opened to a grand new vista. By telling the patient, "I, the doctor, am also on a journey," I become more human, and the barriers begin to fall down.

I do have to be careful that my own interests are not being served at the expense of the patients. I think of it as being the difference between:

A. *"Now let me see how I can feel better by talking to this patient,"* and
B. *"Now let me help this person, and if I can learn something for myself then that is a bonus for me."*

With the latter attitude, I open myself to those encounters that are mutually enriching. I allow for the joyous surprise of synchronicity; I give myself over to God's Time. I truly believe that is what was happening for both me and Dale during the decade of the eighties.

CHAPTER

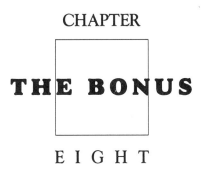

THE BONUS

E I G H T

There have been so many good things for me that have come out of my association with drunks, it just floors me sometimes. One thing has been some good laughs.

There was the elderly mother of one of my middle-aged male alcoholic patients. She was struggling to get the hang of this family recovery business, and especially she was struggling to learn the lingo. When her son had just celebrated his first six months of sobriety, she was telling us with great sincerity how "wonderful it is, he just passed his six-months – uh – what is it? – CELIBACY!" Wow!! that's a tough program we run!

And then there was Cleopatra, Queen of Denial, who after a week in the hospital still claimed her heart was bad and she was really just there for a rest. When I asked her what she thought of the Twelve Steps, she complained that she would rather take the elevator!

Besides laughs, there have been plenty of other bonus points. I should not fail to mention the satisfaction in seeing former patients coming back to sponsor the novices. And a tingle goes up my spine when I hear that one of our most hopeless-appearing roughnecks has earned his one-year AA sobriety chip and shows up at meetings regularly. I used to try and make prognoses when patients left treatment. After several glaring deficiencies in my crystal ball, I have decided that, truly, "God disposes." So I let the chips fall where they may, and as often as not they fall into the hands of those whom some might consider "down for the count." The miracles keep rolling in.

Of all the extra benefits I have received, though, I am particularly thankful for the spinoff from AA recovery that has found its way into my personal life. I could see, as have many others, that the Twelve-Step process has something to say to all of us, alcoholic or not. One of the things that it said to me, very clearly, came out of the "moral inventory" of the Twelve Steps: I needed to make a confession – capital C.

I decided to make my confession in the church, to the priest. I didn't have an AA sponsor or a therapist, those modern-day confessors, so I did it the old-fashioned way. I called Father Murray's office (Emile, the earlier priest in my story, had retired by then) and spoke to his secretary. When Father Murray wasn't immediately available to take my call, I explained the reason for wanting him, that I wished to talk to him about making a confession. There was a pause, then a note of anxiety in the secretary's voice as she explained he would call me back *as soon as possible.* Hannibal Lecter hadn't come on the scene yet, so I'm not sure why she treated this so urgently. She relaxed a little when I explained I wasn't cleaning blood stains from a chain saw or some such, that there was really no emergency.

Fortunately, Father Murray was very understanding of a psychiatrist coming to him, asking to make a first confession. He met with me initially to go over the process, to clarify my expectations, and basically to prepare me for the experience. This was necessary, since I was an Episcopalian and, therefore, a novice penitent, and I welcomed some instruction. He provided written materials to guide my preparations.

I explained to Father Murray that I had been contemplating a formal confession for a year or so. That I felt a need to clean the slate and to seek God's forgiveness through an intermediary. And that the idea had first come to me as I had witnessed the healing effects of the "moral inventory" taken by my alcoholic patients. The guts of the Twelve-Step Program — Steps 4 through 9 — has to do with a sort of confessional. A look at these steps, quoted from the Big Book, will make this clear:*

4. *Made a searching and fearless moral inventory of ourselves.*

5. *Admitted to God, to ourselves, and to another human being the exact nature of our wrongs.*

6. *Were entirely ready to have God remove all these defects of character.*

7. *Humbly asked Him to remove our shortcomings.*

8. *Made a list of all persons we had harmed, and became willing to make amends to them all.*

9. *Made direct amends to such people wherever possible, except when to do so would injure them or others.*

I had seen hundreds of patients work through these steps. I had seen them struggle with the process, resist it, postpone it, and finally complete the steps with great relief. Typically, Step 5 — admitting one's wrongs to another human being — was completed with the

---

* These six steps are reprinted with permission. See the Appendix for a listing of the entire Twelve Steps.

sponsor. Recovering alcoholics brought their lists of immoral incidents and deficiencies to a meeting (or meetings) with their sponsors, their AA mentors and confidants. Paraphrase that: Parishioners bring their litany of sins to a confessional with their priest, who is their spiritual director and confidant.

The parallels were too obvious for me to ignore. It became clear to me that the wisdom of the AA founders and the centuries of practice in Christendom were closely allied. It is not hard to understand this connection, given that Bill Wilson, one of the founders of AA, was heavily influenced by the Oxford Group. (This was a Christian renewal movement with which he had become involved and which had led directly to his turning-point conversion experience.)

At the same time it was beginning to dawn on me that most of us outside of AA are missing something by not participating in such a ritual. We don't have anyone to confess us. True — many who are in psychotherapy do, in a way, confess their "sins" to the therapist. However, the ostensive purpose is more often to clarify problems and understand motives, rather than to find forgiveness and correct moral flaws. So even the small proportion of the population who undergo psychotherapy do not get the full measure of cleansing and redemption offered by the AA moral inventory.

Others may be fortunate enough to have close friends or family — even spouses — with whom they can "tell all." Such intimacy and risk-taking are unusual, however, in the everyday world of relationships. Fear of judgment and betrayed confidentiality generally inhibit this kind of openness.

It might be said that Protestants threw one of the babies out with the bathwater. When certain reformers decided that intermediaries were not necessary with God, they were undoubtedly mostly right. But it seems to me that something very powerful happens in telling one's confession of sins to another human being. There is an accountability in that experience that is different from confession to God in prayer. It is just too easy and routine (speaking for myself), and *anonymous* to pray for forgiveness. It is private and most often silent. This is not to say that personal, private prayer of confession to God is valueless — of course not. But, for me, it lacks something. Person-to-person is more real. Or at least it seems it has the potential for that. Perhaps routine confessions can become rote and meaningless, but I had not come close to that scenario.

Thus it came to pass that I was impressed with the spiritual healing proceeding from this Fifth Step of the AA process, and I took it upon myself to find a confessor. Preparing for this, I used the material Father Murray had provided and followed an outline of transgression categories. I spent a good bit of my spare time over a couple of months, working my way down the list: fifty-four years' worth of mistakes, miscalculations, and misbehavior. I left off the petty stuff, like shoplifting a plastic ruler from the five-and-dime when I was eight years old. Besides, I had paid my dues on that one when my mother discovered it and made me return it, with heartfelt apologies to the sales clerk. I think that was my first and last theft of tangible assets.

I tried to talk myself out of listing the IRS infractions. I mean, is it really possible to sin against the government? To whom would I make amends? A personal apology to all twenty thousand bureaucrats? A compromise came to mind: I would make *one* confession for *all* my peccadillos with Uncle Sam and not try to list all the meals I had written off on medical conventions when my wife's tab was included. The bottom line, though, was that I needed to amend my ways, if not all my prior tax returns.

It was a most difficult, instructive, and potent process, to review a lifetime and pick out those things for which I was truly sorry and to put those on paper in preparation for the formal meeting with my priest.

We followed the liturgy for the Reconciliation of a Penitent from *The Book of Common Prayer*, and about an hour and many tear-stained pages later, I emerged with a sigh of relief and wonder. It had ended so quickly and simply. There was no long dialogue between us, no extemporaneous words of comfort or congratulation. I guess I was accustomed to therapy sessions ending with some of these interactions; some recognition from the therapist, summary of the session, directions for the next session, etc. No, this session ended simply with words of forgiveness. It was so strong that way. Fifty years of rambling error, transgressions that were ordinary to the observer but deadly serious to me, all this wiped clean with the priest's words, "The Lord has put away your sin. Go in peace, and pray for me, a sinner."

I could have kept going through the motions of the AA recovery process with my patients, taken care of their medical needs, and observed what happened. (Needless to say, I had done that a few times in my career.) Yet, if I had not exposed myself in a meaningful way to what that process *meant*, if I had not drawn some conclusions about its relevance for my own life, I would have been much the loser. If I hadn't allowed myself to feel *with* my patients – their joys and sorrows, the moments of quiet surrender, the tearful acknowledgment of love for fellow patients, the surprising joy of being accepted and forgiven – if I had shielded myself and hadn't allowed, at times, my tear-stained face to confront the other one, I would have missed the chance of a lifetime. A chance to grow with my patients. A chance to find a springboard to new insights for myself.

There is nothing particularly novel about these ideas. It is a common observation that all participants in a human encounter are changed to some degree by the experience. The change may be negligible or momentous, or something in-between. The aggregate of these encounters helps to shape our personalities and progression through life. In no small measure, however, the way we approach encounters has something to say about the extent of the impact upon us. That is, if I *expect to learn* from my patients, I will undoubtedly undergo more growth than when I only *expect to effect change* in the patient. In either circumstance, I may be changed as a result, but in the latter case, it will be more or less accidental, unconscious, minimal, and perhaps unwelcome.

Likewise, the idea of applying the Twelve Steps of AA to other life problems is not new. The proliferation of "_____-Anonymous" groups is a formidable phenomenon these last few decades. Their success is a testimony, I believe, to the key human needs that are being met. I am led to ponder the questions:

- What can we "mortals" learn from the Twelve-Step Program?
- What can be borrowed and transplanted into our lives that will allow us to taste the spiritual and emotional fruits of recovery?
- How can we nonalcoholics asssimilate these steps into our everyday living?

When I think about applying recovery principles to my life, I am aware that there are aspects of the healing process of AA that go beyond the Twelve Steps. When I chose to pluck out Steps 4 and 5 and take myself to the confessional chamber, I was selecting only a portion, albeit a mighty important one, of the process. Yet the entire experience includes more than just the Twelve Steps; there are also the meetings and the fellowship to consider.

First, the meetings. We "earth people," as AA members call us, can attend open Twelve-Step meetings, to let it rub off on us. My first such exposure had left me with a clear impression that *honesty,* when manifested in a *trusting, supportive environment* where *love* is in no short supply, is a cleansing, self-affirming experience. I believe we nonalcoholics can find similar, if not identical settings, to AA in which to practice such honesty.

I have most closely experienced the small group experience of Twelve-Step meetings in selected church-related activities; particularly the Cursillo Reunion Group, to which I referred earlier. Although the purpose of that group is clearly *not* therapy, it does offer the ingredients for *spiritual healing;* namely, a small group of people who trust each other, who meet regularly over an extended period of time, and who have a common purpose (in this case, spiritual renewal). We meet weekly to review the prior week's activity; to offer support and, at times, advice; to pray together; and to recommit ourselves to the Christian life. These meetings-with-a-purpose bring a note of accountability to my weekly life that is helpful. Elise participates in this also, and that makes it all the more important to me. And good fortune would have it that my priest/friend, Emile, and his wife, Martha, are also in the group. Martha's library is a never-ending source of new life to me, as I have discovered and rediscovered authors such as Frederick Buechner, C.S. Lewis, and Henri Nouwen.

I might have found a support group in a setting outside of the church. Quite clearly, most therapy groups offer this opportunity, on a fee-for-service basis, but I haven't felt a call to that experience. Even informal, unstructured groups of people, such as may aggregate in a work or community setting or simply as groups of friends, may also approximate this type of support group.

Recently, I have been fortunate enough to participate in such a group of informally structured friends. We simply call it a Men's Group, and we meet monthly at each others' homes. The impetus for this came partly from some of the ideas being formulated by Robert Bly *et al*, popularly referred to as the "Men's Movement." More significantly, however, the group arose simply out of a sense of need: the need to be able to talk seriously with a group of like-minded friends about the things in life that mean the most to us. One of our members put it in a nutshell when he said, "I just can't say what I need to say at a cocktail party; I'd like to be able to be for-real with someone for a change." Dag Hammarskjöld said it quite well, too, in his posthumously-published collection of meditations, *Markings*:

> To be "sociable" – to talk merely because convention forbids silence, to rub against one another in order to create the illusion of intimacy and contact: what an example of la condition humaine. Exhausting, naturally, like any improper use of our spiritual resources. In miniature, one of the many ways in which mankind successfully acts as its own scourge – in the hell of spiritual death.

Here is the bottom line: Small groups – groups that we are drawn to by our own particular values and circumstances, groups in which we can be honest, with people we trust and respect — provide the healing, nurturing environment that we all need.

In addition to the meetings, there is the contribution of the AA fellowship. You might well ask, "Isn't the fellowship the same as the meetings?" The answer is quite clearly, "No." It would be more accurate to say that the meetings provide the opportunity for the fellowship to develop.

"Isn't that what happens when most people get together regularly?" you might counter. "Don't we all gravitate in our social lives to people with whom we feel comfortable and share similar values? What does the AA experience tell us about *fellowship* that doesn't come naturally?"

I believe what is missing most often in our "get togethers" is the special relationship offered by the AA *sponsor*. If you have a best friend, or remember having one from your teen-age years, that person might come close to being sponsor-like. Each AA member is encouraged early on in the Program to get a sponsor, someone who can be an anchor in the storm of recovery. God needs some earthly help. So the AA member has a fleshed-out representative who will talk back. The sponsor comes to be a best friend, advocate, confessor, and therapist, all rolled into one. Instead of having to go up to someone, as you may have in your fifth grade wonderful innocence, and ask, "Will you be my best friend?," you get to ask, "Will you be my sponsor?" That's more palatable for us sophisticated (read: inhibited) adults.

Those of us outside the AA community would do well to find our own sponsor surrogate. This could be a spiritual director through our church, a wise and spiritually mature best friend, or even a spouse. I have two or three friends who fulfill this role in my life, one a clergyman. I find it helpful to bounce things off these friends at selected times, to know that they are available and will listen.

The third element of importance in the AA Program is, of course, the Twelve Steps.* They comprise what I see as four essential elements that we can assimilate into our lives.

Steps 1 through 3 constitute the first element, that of the awesome task of humbling ourselves to the full recognition of our powerlessness over our lives, as long as we remain self-centered and willful. These steps further require that we reach beyond ourselves, to God, for strength and direction in self-renewal. This is the core, the central layer deep within the AA Program that may well be the *sine qua non* of its success. It is the invitation that reaches out to all of us, alcoholic or not.

Steps 4 through 9 constitute the second element, which includes the moral inventory, confession, making amends, and change of character. Wow! After turning things over to God, isn't it supposed to get easier? I'm afraid not. It gets clearer, but not easier. I am sure I have been less than one hundred percent complete in my own confessional, not only with my discrete sins but with persistent character flaws that undergird the wrongful acts: the kudzu patch on my Southern soul. When I find myself a bit complacent, I read the "Litany of Penitence," page 267 of *The Book of Common Prayer* of the Episcopal Church, and there I find many fertile areas for soul-searching. Moreover, after sharing my list of moral indiscretions with another human being (my priest) and with God, I still need to make direct amends.

Asking for forgiveness is tough. I haven't finished this process, by any means, but at least I have started. The first individual I tried it with responded beautifully, and I have made a new friend as a result: He is one of the members of our Men's Group. The next one responded

---

* See the Appendix for a listing of the Twelve Steps.

angrily, partly, I think, because the incident was too fresh and angry feelings too close to the surface. So I will try again with him. I think I have a lifetime project ahead of me.

In fact, this "lifetime" aspect characterizes the third element, made up of Steps 10 and 11. These steps summon the alcoholic to a continuing process of inventory and daily practice of meditation. My memory is so short, and my will so questionable, that I need daily reminders and frequent rituals to keep me on task. I need regular time to meditate, time to take stock of myself. This may be the most challenging part of the process, requiring as it does a self-discipline and ongoing dedication to the principles of recovery. Here is where relapse occurs — whether it is a binge of drinking or a binge of anger. I find it a constant challenge to devote regular time to meditation. Perhaps that is why monastic retreats have such an appeal to me: They provide a setting in which nothing else is expected of me. But there are many styles of daily spiritual disciplines that may be adopted.

This brings me to the final element of recovery from which I think we can learn — the Twelfth Step. This is the step that involves "passing it on" to others. It is like the Great Commission of scriptural fame: "Go ye into all the world . . ." It is the evangelical finale, the reminder that we will keep our salvation only if we share it. In my professional arena, I am reminded that my best times for keeping up with the psychiatric literature have been when I have had responsibility for teaching others. As the line in the song goes, love isn't love until you've given it away.

In my weekly Cursillo Reunion Group, one of the topics of discussion is what we refer to as "Apostolic Action." Each of the group members reports on the previous week's successes or failures in "passing it on," in evangelizing the community around us. Some call it witnessing.

It is the aspect of Christianity that comes hardest for me. I think I like the way AA does it. They work by "attraction," not "promotion." They respond to pleas for help but do not force their dogma on anyone. I may be accused of belonging to "Christians Anonymous," unless I find more freedom in this aspect of my program.

AA folks refer to "twelfth step work" or "twelve stepping it" whenever they are involved in helping another alcoholic into or through recovery. They are always quick to point out that this activity keeps *them* sober, that they are doing it for *themselves*, but I believe that this is only a half truth. Try as they might, their unvarnished altruism raises its beautiful head.

So it was with Bob R., when he was teaching me in his languid manner, by example. So it was with Dale when he shared with me his desperate moments and finally his moments of surrender and acceptance. So it is with all of us, when we reach out to others by intention or by accident – God's "accidents," of course – and thereby help to bring them, and us, to wholeness.

That completes the picture: the meetings, the fellowship, the steps. These gifts and opportunities offered by the AA Program are within reach of all of us. It was up to me to put together my own package that would contain these ingredients. Some would say that I didn't have to look very far to find my gift, all wrapped up with an ecclesiastical ribbon. Most churches would find it hard to disavow many of the essential elements of AA recovery. Indeed, it is true that many alcoholics recover by aligning themselves zealously with a church or denomination without setting foot in an AA meeting place. They either "get religion" or "get AA." Some do both. Most importantly, they do it *with others*. Thomas Merton has said it well in *The Seven Storey Mountain*:

It is a law of man's nature, written into his very
essence and just as much a part of him as the desire
to build houses and cultivate the land and marry and
have children and read books and sing songs, that he
should want to stand together with other men in order
to acknowledge their common dependence on God,
their Father and Creator.

Whether the setting be Roman Catholic, Orthodox, Protestant, Judaic, Hindu, Buddhist, Moslem or Unitarian; whether we seek Heaven, Nirvana, or Enlightenment; whether our hero is Abraham, Mohammed, or Jesus or Bill W.; we find ourselves when we are lost in the company of our spiritual kin.

So be it.

CHAPTER

COMPLETING THE CIRCLE

N I N E

We shall not cease from exploration
And the end of all our exploring
Will be to arrive where we started
And know the place for the first time.

– T.S. Eliot

Psychiatry has evolved from the mists of ancient mysticism into the realm of modern medicine. Hence, you might ask if it isn't regressive to revive spirituality as a vital ingredient in the practice of my specialty. Isn't this throwing us back to primitive times, to the days of medicine men and women, the shaman who invoked gods and cast out demons? Isn't this what happens when I advocate that a psychiatrist work with a patient's spiritual self — not only acknowledging the spiritual dimension as being important in the patient's life outside the consultation room but bringing it into the therapeutic process in a significant way? Is this not undermining all the progress made in psychiatry in the past decades?

I think not.

There are others who would agree. C. G. Jung, for one. From his *Modern Man in Search of a Soul*, the following statement bears testimony to the depth of his appreciation of spiritual principles in healing patients:

> *During the past thirty years, people from all the civilized countries of the earth have consulted me. I have treated many hundreds of patients, the larger number being Protestants, a smaller number Jews, and not more than five or six believing Catholics. Among all my patients in the second half of life — that is to say, over thirty-five — there has not been one whose problem in the last resort was not that of finding a religious outlook on life. It is safe to say that every one of them fell ill because he had lost that which the living religions of every age have given to their followers, and none of them has been really healed who did not regain his religious outlook. This of course has nothing whatever to do with a particular creed or membership of a church.*

Jung is one voice in the wilderness, advocating that we psychiatrists open the door to spiritual dialogue between ourselves and our patients.

It only makes sense to do so. Otherwise, psychiatry is like holistic medicine that has a hole in it. If anyone should treat the whole person, it should be we psychiatrists. Maybe that *is* harking back to primitive healers with only a more high-tech headdress. But I don't mind being called a modern-day shaman. They did (or do) wonderful things for people. Mix a few herbs (prescribe psychopharmaceuticals), chant a few incantations (exhort the patient to a higher level of spiritual function), cast out some demons (allow patient to ventilate), and there you have it. Modern psychiatry. What goes around comes around. The circle is complete.

Nowhere is this better illustrated than on the chemical dependency treatment unit. Nowhere have I seen it work any better than it did with Dale. The unfolding of his adventure (and misadventures) toward and into recovery was a thing of beauty — from the present perspective. At times it was perplexing, frustrating, and, yes, grueling. And yet he and I can now see the necessity, and even purpose, of it all. With Dale, I had to put on my headdress and do the dance. Dale had to live, to survive, until he woke up.

Today Dale believes that his first real spiritual awakening germinated in that shoddy motel room when he was humbled to his knees. It was nurtured through Crestwood and Hazelden, and continues to mature in the program of Alcoholics Anonymous. His journey is very similar to what is described in the Big Book, page 569: "Such a change could hardly have been brought about by himself. What often takes place in a few months could seldom have been accomplished by years of self-discipline."

Dale says he can't understand, let alone try to describe, what happened to him during those months of daily AA meetings — except that he learned the most important thing: He could call on a Higher Power to help him keep away from alcohol. He also became certain that belief in a Higher Power is a *must* for him, and probably for many others, to stay sober.

Recently, as a guest speaker at a local Alcoholics Anonymous meeting, Dale summed up his life story:

Today I'm pleased to be me — who I am, where I am, what I am, and doing what I am — almost all the time. The Big Book says it will get better, and I will testify to that — Amazing Grace.

As Dale looked back on his recovery experience, he could describe it only as a miracle. He continued to be astonished that the AA Program could be so simple and yet have such a workable solution to the problems associated with trying to live a sober, healthy life style.

Only the nagging specter of his brother Curtis' death marred the landscape of this new life. How often he wished Curtis was with him, wished they could have a long — and sober — all-nighter together!

Dale was determined, though, not to sit by and grieve himself into obscurity. Unaccustomed as he was to being idle, it wasn't long before he was generating another career orientation. Let's see — how many would this make for him? Teacher, FBI agent, teacher, juvenile probation officer — what next? He didn't leave me in suspense for very long. After about nine months' sobriety, he announced to me that he wanted to be an addiction counselor. He didn't ask me if it was a good idea; he presented me with his plan to become certified in the field. Some things about Dale hadn't changed, thank God! He still was goal-directed and assertive. It's just that now his aims were loftier, and his drivenness was gone. He was approaching this idea of a new career with a touch of serenity, instead of his prior compulsiveness.

He recalls the germination for the idea starting while he was in treatment at Hazelden:

My roommate and I took long walks, and the subject of our careers often came up. Half seriously, we spoke of becoming counselors. There were plenty of role models around. The staff-to-patient ratio was about one-to-five, so interaction was abundant. I was assigned a "primary therapist" to work with me closely. She was a saintly, compassionate person. My roommate had a different therapist, a retired military man about age sixty with whom I also identified. My new ambitions were founded in this setting of nurturing concern.

When Dale returned to Huntsville, he was not employed, and so he threw himself into the AA Program, attending at least one meeting a day for a year. Soon he was chairing meetings, and his leadership abilities were evident. He spoke well at meetings, telling his story more confidently as the days and months marched on. He found himself being called on to speak frequently, and soon he was doing AA committee work. He found all this immensely important to his growth and development, and, at the same time, he was discovering he had a knack for helping others. He relished Twelve-Step calls to motels at three a.m. Maybe his experience in law enforcement helped him to approach these situations fearlessly. He certainly found joy in this work.

It was quite natural, then, that he would continue to nurture the notion of a career as an addiction counselor. He didn't need the money, but he did need the involvement, and he needed to continue to enhance his own recovery while practicing the Twelve Steps. On a trip back to Minnesota to visit relatives sometime in 1988, he decided to drop by Hazelden to inquire about their counselor training program. He had known of this by its reputation and longed for an opportunity to study at the place where his own healing had begun.

He was disappointed to hear that he would be among two hundred or so on the waiting list for the training program. When he tried to argue that he should be given a chance at it because he was a "graduate," he was then informed that approximately half of the applicants were also former patients! Somewhat discouraged but not disheartened, Dale returned to Huntsville and kept his eyes open for opportunity.

I told him what he already knew: that he was rushing things some, that he would not be hired to work in a treatment program without at least two years' sobriety. No one seems to know whence comes that bit of folk wisdom, the magic two-year dictum, but it is surely fixed in the mind of the treatment industry, and it seems to serve a good purpose.

Many newly recovering individuals become enamored of the idea of counseling careers. It is as natural as youngsters wanting to be a teacher when they have a particularly good experience with one. The treatment encounter is an intensive one, and the relationships forged there are often very close. Patients admire the counselors and may desire to emulate them. Couple this with the enthusiasm accompanying recovery, and you have the makings of a zealous recruit for the treatment profession. Often this is a transient ambition, not much more than a passing fancy. With others, however, the urge is more serious. As with Bob R.

And with Dale. For him, it was a good way to hatch two birds with one egg. Dale could put in productive years that would help solidify his recovery program, and the treatment profession would collect a valuable addition to its ranks.

Not every recovering person is cut out to be a counselor, motivation notwithstanding. There are verbal and interpersonal skills that must be present, in addition to the intellectual requirements of mastering a new field of clinical expertise. Having one's heart in the right place is a necessary but not sufficient condition for the job.

Emotional stability is also important. That's one reason for the two-year wait. The emotional baggage of this disease can wreak havoc on a person. Recovery is a physical, emotional, and spiritual process that takes time. Counselors in this field need to have their act together as much as possible to be able to help others in an accountable manner. Additional psychiatric problems can complicate recovery, so we don't encourage someone who has undiagnosed and untreated major psychiatric problems into a counseling role.

Since Dale was clear on these counts, I didn't try to blow the whistle on him. On the contrary, I gently encouraged him in this new direction. Perhaps it was partly pride of ownership. I felt a real stake in Dale's life at that point, and it was a boost to me to see him with these ambitions. It seemed to me to be a fitting completion to this story.

Sure enough, a few months later Dale was offered a position as part-time counselor assistant (a job not requiring formal training) at — you guessed it — Crestwood Hospital. I came in to make rounds one morning, and there he was, all spit-shined and beaming. He had a note pad in one hand and the Big Book in the other. Armed to the teeth. He was a little nervous, I think, which was good. You don't want to be too cocky in this business, especially if you are a rookie.

Dale initiated his next career by lecturing to groups of patients who were struggling, just as he had, to grasp a thread of hope and begin the long slow climb to recovery. It wasn't difficult for him to empathize. He saw the same raw emotions, the defiance, the physical and emotional wreckage that were a part of his own history.

How did he think he could help them? What did he have to offer?

For one thing, he had his own story to tell; and in telling that story, he didn't need any notes. It was etched into his bones.

For another, he had the AA story to relate. He was plied with outlines to follow, to be sure he covered the necessary material. But it was the stuff he was living by — the Steps — and it was second nature to him.

I saw him at the hospital each day of his first week on duty. Later that same week I got a telephone call from the hospital. My secretary told me it was Dale. I picked up the phone, pushed the lighted button, and wondered if he were going to tell me something like: "Dr. Goodson, this is Dale at Crestwood. We have a new patient for you. He's alcoholic, first time in treatment. I think you'll like him."

CHAPTER

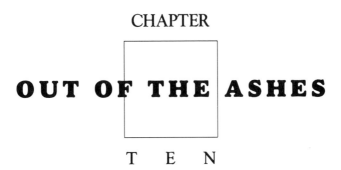

OUT OF THE ASHES

T E N

About the time Dale and I were celebrating his apparent victory over several offerings from the Diagnostic and Statistical Manual of the American Psychiatric Association, I came upon my own encounter with the International Classification of Diseases, specifically Non-Hodgkins Lymphoma, commonly known as cancer of the lymph glands. The good news from Marshall Schreeder, my oncologist, was, "You'll probably live many years"; the bad news, "It can't be cured." This was March 10, 1988. I know the date because I immediately began to keep a journal. There's nothing like cancer to make you start doing some things you've been telling yourself you'll "get around to soon." Like telling certain people you've taken for granted that you love them; like keeping a journal; like writing a book about yourself and a patient.

By March 30th, I had procured a latest-edition copy of *Immunology* by Roitt, Brostoff, and Male, a text recommended by Bob and John Johnson, my old fraternity brothers at Vanderbilt who had taken up specialties I was fast coming to admire: hematology/oncology and immunology, respectively. Since my days in medical school, the field of immunology (and, hence, lymphatic-related cancers) had run away from me. I felt like an old mechanical Underwood in a room full of 386SXs.

Once I decided my doctors probably knew what they were doing — or more likely, that I wouldn't be able to tell whether they did or not — I became their patient and did what they said.

This included such adventures as bone marrow biopsies, universal CT scans, and a trip to Birmingham to see Max Cooper. I had never heard of him prior to this, but clearly I should have. He is one of the premier researchers in lymphatic cancers, and my fortune was that his shop was only a two-hour drive down I-65, at The University of Alabama in Birmingham Medical Center. What he did, roughly speaking, was this: He took my cancer cells and married them to a mouse colony, to maintain a strain that could be manipulated and targeted with monoclonal antibodies and other exotic ammunitions. Then new treatment techniques could be tried out *in vitro* before being used on me, if and when the time comes for pioneer work. No unkind remarks, please, if you notice me twitching my facial whiskers rapidly.

I was fortunate to be selected because this is expensive research and few are chosen. Marshall Schreeder talked Cooper into it by stressing that I would be a good subject: I would show up when I was asked, and I would be willingly to distribute pieces of my organs to his henchmen — er, research fellows. And, more to the point, I had an unusual cancer celltype — biphenotypic, which means there are two derivative cancer cells emanating from a bad old stem cell. It's kind of like having multiple personality: Everyone wants to look at you and study you.

I went through the usual gymnastics of cancer patients: renewing magazines for one year instead of two, converting solid to liquid assets wherever I could, and, in general, avoiding long-term commitments. I also searched for humor wherever I could find it ... like laughing with my father-in-law, who has the same type of cancer, when he refers to us as "lymphomaniacs." Then there were the internal hoops to jump through: Did I really want to live, after all? Wasn't this a good excuse to just give up and die? Why go through old age, decrepitude, senility, more Vanderbilt football? Fifty-two years should be quite enough. They'd been rich and rewarding; my children were all on their own; I had good life insurance and a pension plan for Elise's security.

Deliciously self-indulgent and self-pitying as this trend of thought was, I didn't dwell on that side of the issue for long. I knew down deep I really did want to live. The last few years of my life had seen the turnaround that dictated this conclusion. I had found a new lease on life with an enlivening spiritual burst, and cancer shouldn't — couldn't — squelch that.

I had lots of things going for me, not the least of which were a small group of women in my life — my wife and children — by the names of Elise, Dorothy, Cindy, and Willa; and Dorothy was pregnant with my first grandchild. In addition, I had the example of my father's experience with the same type cancer. Houston Goodson lived sixteen years after his lymphoma was diagnosed, and all but the last three months of his seventy-six years were relatively free of major disability from the disease. His chemotherapy sessions had been inconvenient but not devastating.

I recall with a smile his oft-repeated response to inquiries about his health: "Oh, everybody has to have something, and I've got a little cancer." The tough old politician/fighter had endured it all with class and hardly a complaint. He even broke his neck one time, falling off the roof he was repairing at his lake house. This happened just a couple of years before his death, and he lay helpless in ninety-degree-plus

Alabama heat for several hours before anyone realized something must be wrong and came to the remote cabin. Ironic that he had earlier done such a good job keeping unwanted intruders away from his lake house!

I mention this episode because I believe that was the last drinking episode in my father's alcoholic career. Oh yes, he was alcoholic. You may have guessed that from my earlier references to "hard drinking" in Chapter Five. A few days after his accident at the lake, while he was in a Stryker Frame with half of Ace Hardware's inventory in his skull, I went out to the cabin to check it out and secure it. Sure enough, on the kitchen shelf rested an empty pint bottle of Kentucky Tavern, just as he had left it before tackling the leaky roof.

I looked at the bottle, shook my head in disbelief, and tossed it in the green garbage bag. He had told us of his painful attempts to move himself from the porch into the cabin, to use the phone. I couldn't help but conclude he was really trying to get inside in order to get rid of the evidence. I decided that no one else needed to know about the bottle, at least not then. Certainly my mother didn't need to know. She had suffered enough from Dad's drinking; no need to disabuse her of the notion that he had quit following his stroke a few years ago. So I kept my little secret, not telling Dad I knew until he had recovered enough that I thought he might be relieved to know I was the lone visitor to the cabin. I really felt like giving him the devil, but his condition was too weak for that.

So there I was, the Medical Director of the Crestwood Alcohol and Drug Treatment Unit, a member of the American Academy of Addiction Medicine, working with patients and families daily to confront denial and stop their behaviors that perpetuated the illness ("enabling behaviors," they are called). There I was, the son of an alcoholic who had been enabled to near-death from a fractured cervical spine. And I was still hiding it, protecting people, protecting myself.

I felt a real kinship with Dale and Mary Lou: Dale, as he had watched his brother, Curtis, die an alcoholic suicide; and Mary Lou, as one who had learned the hard way to stop the protection racket.

As with most alcoholics, the "enabling" was not limited to our family. Being a prominent figure in the community is a distinct liability for the alcoholic. Well-meaning people wanted to protect my father, and they did so. Even the highway patrol got into the act. I remember getting a phone call at eleven p.m. or so one night to go see about him. He had run his car off into a plowed field on US Highway 431, on the way home from the lake house. By the time I arrived on the scene, he was joking with the troopers. He was clearly intoxicated and should have been charged with DUI. They all knew him, though, and didn't do so. Sometimes I think the State Troopers must have put extra cars on duty between Huntsville and Guntersville to protect Dad. The Houston Goodson Patrol. If we checked state employment records, we would probably find a large layoff at the time he finally quit drinking.

And most assuredly none of the Huntsville City Police would ever arrest my dad. Through his tours on the City Council, during the growth spurts of the city, he had been responsible for hiring over half the officers! I believe I was even "enabled" a time or two by this circumstance. I can remember an officer looking at my driver's license and saying something like, "Oh, you must be Houston Goodson's son. He hired me as an officer . . . Well . . . Dr. Goodson, I won't ticket you this time, but you be careful, now, and don't be rolling through any more stop signs."

My father's drinking had become progressively worse during the fifties and sixties, after I had moved out of the home. There were very few drinking episodes from my growing-up years that I can recall. The first I ever knew he drank at all was when I was around eleven years old. There was no major event. I simply discovered him drinking alcohol. Prior to that, I had been taught the evils of drink. We had none in the house except for some foul-smelling homemade wine Dad tried to make a couple of years running. He abandoned the effort after a few exploded Mason jars in the closet convinced my mother that the family's lives were at stake. Dad had his talents, but fermentation was not one of them. When I accidentally found him drinking whiskey that day, it was a shocker to me. What I recall is my sense of disbelief mixed with confusion and disappointment. It was one of those moments of myth-shattering that a young man must eventually experience, a moment of pedestal-kicking, a moment of truth.

I was able to ride that one out, however, and a few years of further maturation brought me to a place where I could accept my father's imperfection. He was not drinking daily then, and in fact I don't recall that inebriation was at all a common occurrence, prior to my college days. It wasn't until the later fifties and sixties that the regular pattern emerged. Curiously, he was able to keep this from interfering directly with his city government position. I am told, by those who were close to him at the time, that he never came to a City Council meeting with alcohol on his breath; and, furthermore, that if someone wanted to call a hasty meeting when my father had been drinking, he would refuse to allow it. He somehow had enough judgment to manage this scenario, but it must have been touch-and-go at times.

I believe he took his last drink that hot summer day at the cabin. I feel sad when I think of what it took for him to reach sobriety. And such a short time before cancer finally took him. What would things have been like if he had gotten into treatment, into AA, earlier in his life? What if he and Mother, my sisters Pat and Mary Lou, what if all of us had gotten into recovery? When I see my patients and their families beginning the journey of self-discovery and reaping the benefits in a life of openness and honesty, I am sad for Dad and our family. When I talk to Pat, who took the brunt of his worst drinking for years after her two older siblings had left home, about her particular pain, I am sad for her. When I think of my feeble attempts over the years to talk Dad into treatment, I am angry that I did not take more aggressive action.

After his death, I found myself even more dedicated to helping alcoholics. And when I contracted lymphoma the same as he had, I knew even more so that in a sense I was carrying his life in mine. I had to survive cancer, as he had done for many years, and fulfill a mission he had left undone: a mission of recovery that he had never enjoyed.

I pray that I will do it better this time. The last time I tried to pull off picking up the baton from my fallen father, I had ended up in a fiasco at the Mental Health Center. How can I make it different this time? How can I keep my ego from driving me to another dismal denouement?

I can't answer for sure, of course, because I am in the middle of it. There are all the ingredients for trouble again; namely, a position of authority (director of the chemical dependency unit) from which I could play out a neurotic desire to please my father while covering it with "doing good deeds." My capacity to fool myself has been historically good, so maybe I'm at it again. The fat lady hasn't sung yet, so I have to observe the plot as I see it unfold.

I don't have the lens of hindsight, but I do have some hunches.

For one thing, I've had a sense of closure with Dad. It came very simply and quietly, and fittingly, on his death bed. The decision had been made the day before to disconnect the I·V and let nature take its course. His immune system just didn't have the punch left to fight the infection, and the draining two-month hospital stay that had frustrated a team of excellent physicians was testimony to the inevitable. Several of our family were in his hospital room until the wee hours, pursuing a death watch. Usually one of us was at his side, murmuring soothing words, singing favorite hymns, listening for his barely audible, but coherent, statements or requests.

My turn came, and after ritually reciting the latest Braves' score and speculating as to whether Dale Murphy would have a good year at bat, I leaned over and kissed him on the forehead. I whispered, "Is it okay for me to kiss my dad?" I had never done that before.

He answered, "Oh yes, I always have a kiss for my boy," and puckered his lips.

We all had been trying to reserve our tears for the part of the hospital room away from his bed, but this time it didn't work that way. Mine shamelessly fell on his bedclothes as I realized that he *had* always had a kiss for me, though it never made it past his heart to his lips until then. That old mill-village mentality wouldn't let men kiss men. In fact, I think I had seen him kiss only his grandchildren, and that not very often.

He breathed his last deep, sighing breath an hour or so later, and I thank God for our final exchange. I have had much less reticence hugging my friends and relatives — even patients — since that time. I have a friend, Bob Stewart, who routinely greets his buddies with a bear hug and kisses them on the forehead. It feels okay to me. When it feels right with my patients, especially older ones and alcoholics, we will hug to celebrate small victories in recovery or to seal the therapeutic relationship as the patient is being discharged from the hospital. Very likely, every time I hug a man, my dad is smiling, and the Great Hugs Account Book in the Sky balances a little better.

So, how do I know I am following a truer path this time? It's not easy to define, but I know within myself that I am different, not *driven* to a *mission*. I take things more as they come, shun the limelight, and delight in the small joys of encounters.

... like the meditation by Hammarskjöld that goes, "Be grateful as your deeds become less and less associated with your name, as your feet ever more lightly tread the earth."

... like "One day at a time," or "Take it Easy" that Bob R. first taught me.

... like when I looked up in church one Sunday morning to see Dale and Mary Lou walking to their seats from the communion altar. I knew they were looking for a church home and that they had narrowed it down to our parish and a couple of others. That moment of commonality was more significant to me than any of our many clinical encounters, from the first one at Crestwood to the dismal ones on the psychiatric unit at Huntsville Hospital.

... like my recent return visit to Boston for a medical meeting. During a lunch break from the large ballroom/lecture hall at the Copley Plaza Hotel, I braved the early spring-disguised wintry blast and exited to the curbside. Looking about, my eye immediately caught a large church building on the right. Since I had no particular agenda, I dodged icy spots and found my way to the entrance. "Trinity Episcopal Church" it said, dedicated 1877, architect Henry Hobson Richardson. An organ concert drew me inside. Bach's Fugue in Something Minor was the current rendering, as I quietly sat on a back row, mouth agape at the beauty — yea majesty — of the church. It was Something Major to me. I listened prayerfully and was overwhelmed with nostalgia of a soul — my soul — that had been through the Lost and Found department. My mind scanned back thirty years, and I saw myself and Elise walking these same streets — Dartmouth, Exeter, St. James, Boylston; eating out at the Cafe Budapest on special occasions (fine apple strudel still!). During my psychiatric residency, we had enjoyed Boston, but I had never been in this church, never even noticed it. And now I was counting these few minutes of worship at Trinity as the most meaningful and worthwhile I had spent in the previous twenty-four hours of high-intensity study at the Harvard Course in Geriatric Psychiatry.

That's how I know things are different this time. I see the world with new eyes. I throw away my watch at lunch break and wait for God's Time to direct me to the previously-invisible church. I feel a bond with coworkers — nurses, fellow psychiatrists, counselors, secretaries — that is more forgiving. I hope they would all say that, too; and a few have from time to time. I think I have less of my *self* to cloud the view of the *other* (patient, colleague, friend, family).

There's still plenty of self to work on, though, and I know that better than anyone. I still have anxieties that dog me from time to time. I find conflict hard to deal with and still get caught up in the pressure to perform well. Cancer hasn't lured my old-brain limbic system from its habitual concerns, and I haven't reached a buddha-like composure, by any means. I'm just different than I was, and I can face each day with that knowledge.

I am grateful that the death threat of the big "C" came at a time when my spiritual soil was prepared and enriched. The garden is better tended now, so weeds are not the threat they might have been. Things seem to fall into place in a timely manner. Even the financial security of my family has been assured in a bizarre way.

In the depths of my worst moments — in fact, about the time I first met Dale in 1980 — the prospects of living very much longer didn't particularly appeal to me. With that in mind, I took out a substantial life insurance policy, just in case things got bad enough. Well ...things *didn't* get bad enough, but I was fortunately stuck with the premiums on this universal life policy recommended by my insurance agent, Jim McCown. Years later, I am thanking Jim for setting me up nicely when he did. He would be sorely challenged to find a policy for me now. Of course, he never knew the reason why Bill Goodson, high school classmate of his wife, Jeanne, and long-term acquaintance, was suddenly coming to him for more life insurance. An act of bleakness has turned into an actual blessing.

Not all of the twists and turns have been auspicious, however. Ironically, about the same time, I played the role of Scotty Templeton in a local community theater production of "Tribute," a play by Bernard Slade. Scotty (played by Jack Lemmon on Broadway and in the movie) is a middle-aged comedian/writer who contracts a *lymphatic cancer* (yes!) and has to do some fancy footwork to bring his life together. That was some three years before I contracted the same illness. Foreshadowing carried to its ridiculous extremity, don't you think? The depression I fell into immediately after that performance was eerie, so much so that I stacked my scripts up on the shelf and haven't trod any boards since that ominous thespian outing. I'm not going to take a chance on getting cast as Willie Loman next time.

Other ironies are more pleasant to report. Like a few years ago when my L4-L5 segments and the cruciate ligament of my right knee made the final pronouncement that tennis and basketball were history for me. This, coupled with the aforementioned theatrical finale, brought me down a few shades on the blue spectrum. Then, out of the blue, an opportunity came in the shape of Charlie McClary, yet another of my old Vanderbilt connections. Charlie and I are among a group who devotedly return to Nashville each October for the Homecoming reunion. On one of these masochistic gridiron adventures, Charlie passed along a challenge having to do with his new-found, treasured sport of bicycling: something to the effect that he bet I couldn't come to Bloomington, Indiana, that next October and finish the "Hilly Hundred," an annual bicycle touring extravaganza in his hometown. I hadn't been on a bike in decades, but the challenge intrigued me.

Before long I was waiting for the first of many catalog orders from *Bike Nashbar* and *Performance* to arrive in the mail. Several hundred miles later I was riding in the pack of the Hilly Hundred, smiling through the pain. Soon I had joined with other guys who found themselves either at a similar stage of ligamentous deterioration or trying to avoid such, and the low-impact, high aerobic sport of bicycling caught on. Importantly, this was not *competitive* bicycling (no racing, please) but just good fun. Since then I have pedaled and coasted away countless hours with Bob Stewart, Dave Barnhart, Tom Tenbrunsel, Charlie, and others, on back roads in Alabama, Indiana, Tennessee, Kentucky, North Carolina, and New England, finding camaraderie with good friends and with nature. Also, finding lessons for living, such as the profound impression that one does not truly appreciate riding *with* the wind until one has ridden *against* it. And that a steep downhill can be intense but evanescent, compared to a long, gentle grade that invites sensory arousal but not adrenalization. My new-found recreation has brought unexpected blessings.

The tapestry of my life continues to be woven. My vantage point now, as always, is on the frayed edge, looking back at the intricately meshed pattern and ahead at the loose threads. I see a long traversing strand that is solid and bold – that of my father, I presume. Then there is another, more subtle strand woven throughout if I look carefully – my mother's. About a third of the way through the woven cloth, a dominant new group of threads picks up: those of family, friends, mentors; of ideas begotten of Vanderbilt and Boston. Then the colors flash and fade chaotically for a piece. There I find a rough-looking thread that has a faint odor of cigar – must be Bob R.! The segment next to the present is rich with color and harmony, blending as it does the lives of Dale and my other patients, my church family, the Cursillo Reunion Group, Men's Group, bicycling companions, my Trappist brothers at Gethsemani. The newest stitches, clean and fresh, are my new grandchildren.

I can't wait to see what the Weaver has in mind for the rest of the cloth. Take that back – I *can* wait. That's what I have learned to do. I've had many second- and third-chances, including surviving a round of chemotherapy; so every day is a gift that I open to see what's inside. I've found that the best things can sometimes come from what seem to be the worst. I'd best not pre-judge the next few rows of stitches in my life.

Out of the ashes rises the new city. Dale and I have discovered this in our own ways. It is an incredible miracle that he lived through all he did. Even from just the standpoint of the hours he spent behind the wheel going to and from work, loaded, it's a miracle. And then there were his blind-drunk forays to Mexico or God-knows-where. If accidents wouldn't claim him, deliberate death surely could have. He carried an aura of suicidality about him, what with his black depressions and eventual psychotic states. God stayed the hand of the grim reaper and let me lend a hand. I was along for the ride, trying to stay one step ahead but usually just barely catching up with Dale's fluctuating clinical state.

Dale came back to life to carry on where his brother, Curtis, could no more. He eventually went back to his Lutheran roots (not the Episcopal church), and he and Mary Lou have settled in at the St. Mark's Lutheran Church in Huntsville. Curtis would have liked that.

As for me, while I was discovering Dale's psychopathology, I was inadvertently finding some of my own. Not that I was alcoholic, or bipolar, or any standard category. I needed an ophthalmologist. Mine was a blind spot, an "I" disorder. Prior to Dale's era in my professional career, it was I who had to cure the patient, I who had to have the answers, I who couldn't "let go and let God." My blind spot was the lack of a spiritual dimension in my life, in my work, in my relationships with my patients, in not allowing things to happen by intuition and God's grace.

With Dale's help, this has changed. Not that other patients haven't also had an impact on me. My encounter with Dale has not accounted for all my spiritual awakenings, but my experience with him was extraordinary and has left an indelible mark on me. I continue to find life in helping to bring sobriety to men and women, people like my father; they don't know it, but they are getting well for him, too.

I guess I have failed to mention that Dale bears a physical resemblance to my dad.

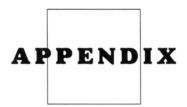

APPENDIX

THE TWELVE STEPS OF ALCOHOLICS ANONYMOUS[*]

1. We admitted we were powerless over alcohol — that our lives had become unmanageable.

2. Came to believe that a Power greater than ourselves could restore us to sanity.

3. Made a decision to turn our will and our lives over to the care of God *as we understood Him.*

4. Made a searching and fearless moral inventory of ourselves.

5. Admitted to God, to ourselves, and to another human being the exact nature of our wrongs.

6. Were entirely ready to have God remove all these defects of character.

7. Humbly asked Him to remove our shortcomings.

8. Made a list of all persons we had harmed, and became willing to make amends to them all.

9. Made direct amends to such people wherever possible, except when to do so would injure them or others.

10. Continued to take personal inventory and when we were wrong promptly admitted it.

11. Sought through prayer and meditation to improve our conscious contact with God *as we understood Him,* praying only for knowledge of His will for us and the power to carry that out.

12. Having had a spiritual awakening as the result of these steps, we tried to carry this message to alcoholics, and to practice these principles in all our affairs.

---

* The Twelve Steps are reprinted with permission of Alcoholics Anonymous World Services, Inc. Permission to reprint portions of this material does not mean that AA has reviewed or approved the contents of this publication, nor that AA agrees with the views expressed herein. AA is a program of recovery from alcoholism — use of the Twelve Steps in connection with programs and activities which are patterned after AA, but which address other problems, does not imply otherwise.

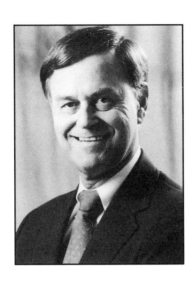

ABOUT THE AUTHOR
William H. Goodson, Jr.

William Goodson is a psychiatrist in private practice in Huntsville, Alabama. Also a certified addiction medicine specialist, he has been medical director of the chemical dependency treatment unit at Crestwood Hospital in Huntsville since 1979. Prior to that he was Director of the Huntsville-Madison County Mental Health Center.

Dr. Goodson and his wife, Elise, who is a middle-school teacher, belong to the Episcopal Church of the Nativity, where they are active in parish life.

His formal higher education was obtained at Vanderbilt University and at Harvard-affiliated hospitals in Boston. But he believes that his best education has come from daily contact with patients and coworkers.

His patient, Dale J., is a former FBI agent who also lives in Huntsville, with his wife, Mary Lou. She has recently retired from her nursing position at Huntsville Hospital.

Other LuraMedia Publications

BANKSON, MARJORY ZOET

Braided Streams:
Esther and a Woman's Way of Growing

Seasons of Friendship:
Naomi and Ruth as a Pattern

"This Is My Body. . .":
Creativity, Clay, and Change

BOHLER, CAROLYN STAHL

Prayer on Wings: *A Search for Authentic Prayer*

DOHERTY, DOROTHY ALBRACHT
and McNAMARA, MARY COLGAN

Out of the Skin Into the Soul:
The Art of Aging

GEIGER, LURA JANE

and PATRICIA BACKMAN

Braided Streams Leader's Guide

and SUSAN TOBIAS

Seasons of Friendship Leader's Guide

GOODSON, WILLIAM (with Dale J.)

Re-Souled: *Spiritual Awakenings of a Psychiatrist
and his Patient in Alcohol Recovery*

JEVNE, RONNA FAY

It All Begins With Hope:
Patients, Caretakers, and the Bereaved Speak Out

and ALEXANDER LEVITAN

No Time for Nonsense:
Getting Well Against the Odds

KEIFFER, ANN

Gift of the Dark Angel: *A Woman's Journey
through Depression toward Wholeness*

LODER, TED

Eavesdropping on the Echoes:
Voices from the Old Testament

Guerrillas of Grace:
Prayers for the Battle

Tracks in the Straw:
Tales Spun from the Manger

Wrestling the Light:
Ache and Awe in the Human-Divine Struggle

MEYER, RICHARD C.

One Anothering:
Biblical Building Blocks for Small Groups

MILLETT, CRAIG

In God's Image:
Archetypes of Women in Scripture

PRICE, H.H.

Blackberry Season:
A Time to Mourn, A Time to Heal

RAFFA, JEAN BENEDICT

The Bridge to Wholeness:
A Feminine Alternative to the Hero Myth

Dream Theatres of the Soul:
*Empowering the Feminine through
Jungian Dreamwork*

SAURO, JOAN

Whole Earth Meditation:
Ecology for the Spirit

SCHAPER, DONNA

Stripping Down:
The Art of Spiritual Restoration

WEEMS, RENITA J.

Just a Sister Away: *A Womanist Vision
of Women's Relationships in the Bible*

I Asked for Intimacy: *Stories of Blessings,
Betrayals, and Birthings*

The Women's Series

BORTON, JOAN

Drawing from the Women's Well:
Reflections on the Life Passage of Menopause

CARTLEDGE-HAYES, MARY

To Love Delilah:
Claiming the Women of the Bible

DUERK, JUDITH

Circle of Stones:
Woman's Journey to Herself

I Sit Listening to the Wind:
Woman's Encounter within Herself

**O'HALLORAN, SUSAN and
DELATTRE, SUSAN**

The Woman Who Lost Her Heart:
A Tale of Reawakening

RUPP, JOYCE

The Star in My Heart:
Experiencing Sophia, Inner Wisdom

SCHNEIDER-AKER, KATHERINE

God's Forgotten Daughter:
*A Modern Midrash: What If
Jesus Had Been A Woman?*

**LuraMedia, Inc. , 7060 Miramar Rd., Suite 104, San Diego, CA 92121
Call 1-800-FOR-LURA for information about bookstores or ordering.**
Books for Healing and Hope, Balance and Justice.